Ethical Concerns in Sport Governance

Sport governance no longer stirs public opinion only when scandals surface; it has become a persistent concern for a number of stakeholders, such as the media, sport followers, and corporates that produce and sponsor sport. Contemporary sport governance is characterised by tension between sport's potential for commercial benefit on the one hand and moral education and social development on the other. The perceived incompatibility of these two aspects has led to intense conversations in the media, administrative circles, and the public sphere about the need for ethics to be the key element of governance. The chapters in this volume explore the contemporary forms of governance that are structured by sport's extensive transnational networks, shifts in what the stakeholders mentioned above understand by 'ethics', and the emergence of new stakeholders. They identify as the two major directions of contemporary sport governance the growing significance of the non-West, especially in relation to event hosting, and the need for controlling the behaviour of emergent interest groups. The latter is a complex constellation of athletes, officials, supporters, lawyers, and politicians who share power and collectively determine corporate and non-profit governance, legal aspects, and regulatory mechanisms from within their subjective locations.

The chapters in this book were originally published in a special issue of *Sport in Society*.

Souvik Naha is a Guest Lecturer in History at West Bengal State University, Kolkata, India. He has edited *Global and Transnational Sport: Ambiguous Border, Connected Domains* (2018) and, with Kausik Bandyopadhyay and Shakya Mitra, *FIFA World Cup and Beyond: Sport, Culture, Media and Governance* (2018). He is the editor of *Soccer & Society*.

David Hassan has published 15 books and 175 other research outputs. He was awarded a Distinguished Research Fellowship from Ulster University, UK in recognition of his outstanding contribution to research. He has held several leadership roles at the university, including Head of School, Head of Research Graduate School, Provost of the Belfast and Jordanstown campuses, and Associate Dean of the Faculty of Life and Health Sciences (Global Engagement).

Sport in the Global Society: Contemporary Perspectives
Series Editor: Boria Majumdar, University of Central Lancashire, UK

The social, cultural (including media), and political study of sport is an expanding area of scholarship and related research. While this area has been well served by the *Sport in the Global Society* series, the surge in quality scholarship over the last few years has necessitated the creation of *Sport in the Global Society: Contemporary Perspectives*. The series will publish the work of leading scholars in fields as diverse as sociology, cultural studies, media studies, gender studies, cultural geography and history, political science, and political economy. If the social and cultural study of sport is to receive the scholarly attention and readership it warrants, a cross-disciplinary series dedicated to taking sport beyond the narrow confines of physical education and sport science academic domains is necessary. *Sport in the Global Society: Contemporary Perspectives* will answer this need.

Recent titles in the series include:

New Perspectives on Association Football in Irish History
Going beyond the "Garrison Game"
Edited by Conor Curran and David Toms

Major Sporting Events
Beyond the Big Two
Edited by John Harris, Fiona Skillen and Matthew McDowell

Research Methodologies and Sports Scholarship
Edited by James Skinner and Terry Engelberg

Sport and Disability
From Integration Continuum to Inclusion Spectrum
Edited by Florian Kiuppis

Ethical Concerns in Sport Governance
Edited by Souvik Naha and David Hassan

Global Markets and Global Impact of Sports
SportsWorld
Edited by John Nauright and Sarah Zipp

Ethical Concerns in Sport Governance

Edited by
Souvik Naha and David Hassan

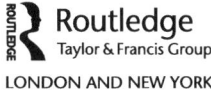

LONDON AND NEW YORK

First published 2019
by Routledge
2 Park Square, Milton Park, Abingdon, Oxon, OX14 4RN, UK

and by Routledge
52 Vanderbilt Avenue, New York, NY 10017

First issued in paperback 2020

Routledge is an imprint of the Taylor & Francis Group, an informa business

© 2019 Taylor & Francis

British Library Cataloguing-in-Publication Data
A catalogue record for this book is available from the British Library

ISBN 13: 978-0-367-58672-0 (pbk)
ISBN 13: 978-1-138-31931-8 (hbk)

Typeset in Minion Pro
by codeMantra

Publisher's Note
The publisher accepts responsibility for any inconsistencies that may have arisen during the conversion of this book from journal articles to book chapters, namely the possible inclusion of journal terminology.

Disclaimer
Every effort has been made to contact copyright holders for their permission to reprint material in this book. The publishers would be grateful to hear from any copyright holder who is not here acknowledged and will undertake to rectify any errors or omissions in future editions of this book.

Contents

Citation Information

The chapters in this book were originally published in the journal *Sport in Society*, volume 21, issue 5 (May 2018). When citing this material, please use the original page numbering for each article, as follows:

Introduction
Introduction: ethical concerns in sport governance
Souvik Naha and David Hassan
Sport in Society, volume 21, issue 5 (May 2017) pp. 721–723

Chapter 1
Beyond governance: the need to improve the regulation of international sport
Jean-Loup Chappelet
Sport in Society, volume 21, issue 5 (May 2017) pp. 724–734

Chapter 2
Sport and politics in a complex age
David Hassan
Sport in Society, volume 21, issue 5 (May 2018) pp. 735–744

Chapter 3
Sport mega-events, the 'non-West' and the ethics of event hosting
Suzanne Dowse and Thomas Fletcher
Sport in Society, volume 21, issue 5 (May 2018) pp. 745–761

Chapter 4
Gulf autocrats and sports corruption: a marriage made in heaven
James M. Dorsey
Sport in Society, volume 21, issue 5 (May 2018) pp. 762–772

Chapter 5
Towards responsible policy-making in international sport: reforming the medical-scientific commissions
Bruce Kidd
Sport in Society, volume 21, issue 5 (May 2018) pp. 773–787

Chapter 6

Canada 2015: perceptions and experiences of the organisation and governance of the Women's World Cup
Carrie Dunn
Sport in Society, volume 21, issue 5 (May 2018) pp. 788–799

Chapter 7

'Trust me I am a Football Agent'. The discursive practices of the players' agents in (un)professional football
Seamus Kelly and Dikaia Chatziefstathiou
Sport in Society, volume 21, issue 5 (May 2018) pp. 800–814

Chapter 8

Motorsport volunteerism: a form of social contract?
David Hassan and Chris Harding
Sport in Society, volume 21, issue 5 (May 2018) pp. 815–832

For any permission-related enquiries please visit:
http://www.tandfonline.com/page/help/permissions

Notes on Contributors

Jean-Loup Chappelet is a Professor of Public Management in the Swiss Graduate School of Public Administration (IDHEAP) at the University of Lausanne, Switzerland. He was the IDHEAP Dean from 2003 to 2011. He is the General Secretary of the International Coubertin Committee and a member of the World Anti-Doping Agency (WADA)'s social science working group and a former member of its education committee.

Dikaia Chatziefstathiou is a Reader in Olympic Studies and the Social Analysis of Sport at Canterbury Christ Church University, UK. Her research interests are in Olympic studies (Olympic Games, Olympic movement, Olympism, and related areas such as Olympic education), globalisation and sport, and sport and culture.

James M. Dorsey is a Senior Fellow at the S. Rajaratnam School of International Studies (RSIS) at Nanyang Technological University, Singapore. He focuses on political and social change in the Middle East and North Africa, the impact of change in the Middle East and North Africa on Southeast and Central Asia and the nexus of sports, and politics and society in the Middle East and North Africa and Asia.

Suzanne Dowse is the Programme Director for the Sport and Health Management and Event Management Degrees at Canterbury Christ Church University, UK. Her teaching specialisms and subject expertise include research methods, international relations and sport, and the political and social implications of hosting sport events.

Carrie Dunn has taught all around the UK, delivering modules on cultural studies, media, and sociology. Her research interests include fandom, sport, feminism, and the consumption of popular culture. As a freelance journalist, she writes for publications including *The Times* and *The Guardian*, and as a broadcaster she is a regular contributor to BBC Radio, Sky News, LBC, and CNN. She has covered events from the Olympics to the Ashes.

Thomas Fletcher is a Senior Lecturer within the Carnegie Faculty at Leeds Beckett University, UK. He specialises in the social and cultural aspects of sport, leisure, and events. His current research interests are broadly related to the sociology of sport and leisure and include 'race'/ethnicity, social identities, heritage, and equity and diversity.

Chris Harding is a PhD Candidate, researching volunteerism in motorsport at the Sport and Exercise Sciences Research Institute at Ulster University, Coleraine, UK. He specialises in contracts management – railways, metro, airports, transportation, complex multidisciplinary projects, international contracts – FIDIC, and contract negotiation – claims & dispute resolution.

NOTES ON CONTRIBUTORS

David Hassan has published 15 books and 175 other research outputs. He was awarded a Distinguished Research Fellowship from Ulster University, UK in recognition of his outstanding contribution to research. He has held several leadership roles at the university, including Head of School, Head of Research Graduate School, Provost of the Belfast and Jordanstown campuses, and Associate Dean of the Faculty of Life and Health Sciences (Global Engagement).

Seamus Kelly is a College Lecturer in the School of Public Health, Physiotherapy, and Population Science at University College Dublin, UK. He has lectured on the BSc, MSc, and Diploma in Sport and Exercise Management programmes since 2002. In terms of research, gaining access to the closed world of professional football was due, in part, to his previous professional and semi-professional playing experience.

Bruce Kidd is a Professor in the Faculty of Kinesiology and Physical Education and the Warden of Hart House at the University of Toronto, Canada. In December 2014, he was appointed as the tenth principal of the University of Toronto Scarborough, Canada. He is an honorary member of the Canadian Olympic Committee and volunteer chair of the Selection Committee, Canada's Sports Hall of Fame.

Souvik Naha is a Guest Lecturer in History at West Bengal State University, Kolkata, India. He has edited *Global and Transnational Sport: Ambiguous Border, Connected Domains* (2018) and, with Kausik Bandyopadhyay and Shakya Mitra, *FIFA World Cup and Beyond: Sport, Culture, Media and Governance* (2018). He is the editor of *Soccer & Society*.

Introduction: ethical concerns in sport governance

Souvik Naha and David Hassan

Sport governance no longer stirs public opinion only when scandals surface; it has become a persistent concern for a number of stakeholders. A combination of the inexorable presence of the media, people's scepticism of those who run their favourite sports, and vagaries of the moral economy of global sport capitalism since the late twentieth century has made governance a newsworthy, momentous and meaningful aspect of elite sports. The media has been attentive to the financial irregularities, the struggles for recognition, and the political and exploitative aspects of sport governance that have come to light rather frequently since the beginning of the twenty-first century. It has played a critical role in shaping sport governance too, especially after the advent of televised sport, sponsorship and marketing. Television forms the economic backbone of modern sport, and digital platforms are set to revolutionize sport coverage. Secondly, sport followers, who double as consumers of media content, understand the challenges of governing what has transformed in the twentieth century from local leisure cultures to highly capitalized industries with a global reach. Depending on their level of interest, they track governance of local clubs, national teams, international federations and similar entities. They are usually aware of the structures of power and ownership, policy-making at various levels, and violation of accountability. Finally, sport administrators, who are drawn from state representatives and the commercial elite operating in both national and transnational contexts, are obliged to run the show, maximize profit and connect with supporters. With the exception of the Middle Eastern monarchies and a few other authoritarian states, sport administrators often subject themselves to self-regulatory measures in order to be legitimized as custodians of the game. Ethical practice is probably one of the most important catechism they encounter at a quotidian level, as transparency and incorruptibility are widely considered necessary attributes of sport governance. The media and sport followers are no exception to the rule of ethics as stakeholders of governance.

This simplified account of the contemporary landscape of sport governance illustrates the tension between the characterizations of sport as a commercial activity and as a mechanism for moral education and social development. The perceived incompatibility of these two aspects has led to intense conversations in the media, administrative circles and the public sphere about the need for ethical concerns to be the key element of governance. The transformation of sport governance from organizing friendly matches to activities ranging from hosting 10,000 athletes and 500,000 tourists during a mega event to determining gender of athletes, has complicated the connotations of administration. Governance, as Hassan and Hamil acknowledge (2010, 343), has overgrown the pattern of club owners hiring athletes and rewarding them for delivering success with little concern for profit maximization. The 'relatively benign business approach' has dramatically changed into an industry-oriented model that contends with problems of racism, doping, match-fixing and money laundering to name a few. The undoing of sport's amateur connections is now a foregone conclusion. The dynamics of revenue generation and redistribution, labour market sustainment, social responsibility, and outreach programmes constantly transform the practice of governance as well as ethics. The reception of Western sports in non-Western regions and the emergence of new sporting endeavours such as e-sports, have appeared to rework the understanding of participation and organization. New expectations and liabilities pose fundamental challenges to the balance of politics and ethics.

The history of FIFA exhibits the complexity of contemporary sport governance like no other entity. As Tomlinson (2014) remarked, it would be incorrect to think of the early presidents as idealist and the latter ones as dictatorial and unaccountable. However, allegations of corruption have escalated, the lack of ethical considerations exposed, and the crisis of integrity heightened since the 2000s, making malpractices from half a century before look like innocuous mistakes. How does one make sense of the shifting underpinnings of ethics in sport governance by inter- and supranational institutions? Many researchers have addressed the governance question in recent times, pondering social capital (Groeneveld, Houlihan, and Ohl 2011), club football (Hassan and Hamil 2011), corporate responsibility (Segaert et al. 2012), national contexts (O'Boyle and Bradbury 2013), and concepts and practices, global order, body enhancement, and sport for development (Auwele, Cook, and Parry 2016). A conference was organized in Oxford in June 2016 to discuss the inclinations of stakeholders as borne out by current tendencies in policy-making, out of which materialized this collection. The participants deliberated the forms of governance emerging from the aggregation of transnational networks, the shifting metonymies of ethical concern and new stakeholder identification. The two major directions of contemporary sport governance identified were the growing significance of the non-West, especially in relation to event hosting, and the need for controlling the behaviour of emergent interest groups. The latter is a complex constellation of athletes, officials, supporters, lawyers, and politicians who share power and collectively determine corporate and non-profit governance, legal aspects, and regulatory mechanisms from within their subjective locations.

The collection opens with Jean-Loup Chappelet's article that ponders the need for administrators to embrace the relevant characteristics of both corporate and democratic governance, and develop international cooperation between state and private actors. David Hassan analyses the fissures between sport's democratizing rhetoric and its increasing appropriation by authoritarian regimes in their quest for respectability. Susan Dowse and Thomas Fletcher complicate the politics of event hosting and power relations between the traditional arbiters and the developing nations. James Dorsey explores the influence of non-Western actors in global sport governance with reference to the Gulf States. While this set of articles interrogate the ethics of decision-making and hierarchy of governance in international sport, the next set examines specific issues that require greater regulation. Bruce Kidd discusses the disputed scientific and ethical substructures of the 'gender eligibility' tests conducted by the IOC and IAAF's medical commission. Carrie Dunn reviews the fan experience of the

2015 FIFA Women's World Cup, identifying the nature of sexism at various levels of football governance. Seamus Kelly and Dikaia Chatziefstathiou look into the alleged unethical behaviour of sport agents and the consequences of their growing influence on club football. Finally, David Hassan and Chris Harding use social contract theory to examine the strategies of recruiting and retaining volunteers for motorsport. The articles recognize that the reinvention of the ethical standards of governance entails fresh challenges and the need for administrators to take up new priorities and responsibilities. This collection looks at the extent and nature of ethical concerns for the new directions in governance.

Disclosure statement

No potential conflict of interest was reported by the authors.

References

Auwele, Y. V., E. Cook, and J. Parry, eds. 2016. *Ethics and Governance in Sport: The Future of Sport Imagined*. Abingdon: Routledge.

Groeneveld, M., B. Houlihan, and F. Ohl, eds. 2011. *Social Capital and Sport Governance in Europe*. Abingdon: Routledge.

Hassan, D., and S. Hamil. 2010. "Models of Football Governance and Management in International Sport." *Soccer & Society* 11 (4): 343–353.

Hassan, D., and S. Hamil, eds. 2011. *Who Owns Football? Models of Football Governance and Management in International Sport*. Abingdon: Routledge.

O'Boyle, I., and T. Bradbury, eds. 2013. *Sport Governance: International Case Studies*. Abingdon: Routledge.

Segaert, B., M. Theeboom, C. Timmerman, and B. Vanreusel, eds. 2012. *Sports Governance, Development and Corporate Responsibility*. Abingdon: Routledge.

Tomlinson, A. 2014. "The Supreme Leader Sails on: Leadership, Ethics and Governance in FIFA." *Sport in Society: Cultures, Commerce, Media, Politics* 17 (9): 1155–1169.

Beyond governance: the need to improve the regulation of international sport

Jean-Loup Chappelet

ABSTRACT

Governance has been a prominent word in international sport circles since the beginning of the twenty-first century. However, better governance will not cure all the ills of this wide-ranging sector and its numerous governing bodies, many of which, including the International Olympic Committee (IOC), the Fédération Internationale de Football Association (FIFA) and the International Association of Athletics Federations (IAAF), have been shaken by corruption. This paper discusses the need for a new approach to sports governance that combines aspects of both corporate and democratic governance. It also shows that combating problems such as doping, match-fixing, hooliganism and sport corruption requires a wider international legal framework, developed through cooperation between government authorities and the sports sector. Only international regulation will ensure sport gains the improved governance it needs in order to preserve its integrity and value in the eyes of the public.

Introduction

It is now almost two decades since people started talking about governance in the Olympic system. The word first caught on in the world of sport during the 'Salt Lake City scandal', which shook the International Olympic Committee (IOC) at the end of 1998 and throughout 1999 (Wenn, Barney, and Martyn 2011). The outcry over inducements paid to several IOC members by Salt Lake City's 2002 Winter Olympics bid committee led the IOC to profoundly reform its governance (Chappelet 2012). Since then, many of the international sport federations (IFs) within the Olympic system have been tarnished by corruption scandals of varying degrees of seriousness. Most recently, in 2015 and 2016, it has been the turn of two of the world's biggest IFs, the Fédération Internationale de Football Association (FIFA) and the International Association of Athletics Federations (IAAF) to be hit by scandal. Since the beginning of the twenty-first century, governmental and intergovernmental bodies, national and international sport governing bodies and academics have put forward numerous lists – more than 30 in total – of governance principles for sport organizations. However, scandals have continued to emerge. Nevertheless, the FIFA and IAAF scandals appear to have been a turning point.

The present article shows that preoccupations referred to under the term governance need to be examined from a much wider perspective, that of the regulation of international sport. Although international sport has its critics, it is a vitally important area that has a unique ability to promote peaceful coexistence and cooperation between people and countries. I begin this paper by presenting the current situation in sports governance. I then outline four possible scenarios for monitoring this governance and discuss three important governance questions that are rarely addressed. Section three describes a theoretical model of governance in which state supervision is a key component in improving the regulation of international sport. The paper concludes with a proposal for a long-term solution for introducing the regulation international sport needs in order to preserve its integrity and socio-educational value in the eyes of the public.

The state of sports governance

Following the Salt Lake City scandal, which led to the expulsion or resignation of ten IOC members in 1999 (and warnings for another ten), several international sport federations have been shaken by revelations of corruption. For example, between 2004 and 2008, the presidents of the IFs for volleyball (FIVB), judo (IJF) and taekwondo (WTU) had to resign both their federation presidencies and their seats on the IOC. Since then, many other 'affairs', some better known than others, have come to light in other IFs, including boxing (AIBA), cycling (UCI), handball (IHF) and weightlifting (IWF), to name just the Olympic federations. Most recently, it has been the turn of the football (FIFA), athletics (IAAF) and shooting (ISSF) federations to be racked by scandal (AFP 2015). These 'affairs' and 'scandals' often result in a change of president.

Although these issues receive little media attention unless they affect a 'major' sport such as football, athletics or cycling, they have resulted in experts and academics taking a close interest in the governance of sport organizations. Hence, the European Union included a list of principles of 'good governance' for the sports movement in its 'Declaration of Nice' in 2000, (EU 2000) and, in January 2001, at a conference on governance held in Brussels by the European Olympic Committees and the International Automobile Federation, Jacques Rogge launched his bid for the IOC presidency by highlighting his position on governance: 'Since Sport is based on ethics and competition on fair play, the governance of sport must comply with the highest standards in terms of transparency, democracy and accountability' (EOC 2001). The research community also made a substantial contribution. For example, Henry and Lee (2004) suggested seven principles for sports governance: Transparency, Accountability, Democracy, Social Responsibility, Equity, Effectiveness and Efficiency. In fact, 35 lists of governance principles had been published by 2013 (Chappelet and Mrkonjic 2013), not including the list published that year by the European Union (EU 2013).

There is now a general consensus that sports governance should combine elements of corporate governance, as applied in the business world (Mallin 2011), and democratic governance, as advocated for the public sector, most notably by the World Bank (Bevir 2010). In fact, sport organizations blend certain characteristics of commercial organizations (especially when they sell broadcasting or marketing rights for their events) with those of public organizations (when they draw up rules for their sports and their events).

In addition to this consensus on the general outline of sport governance (Figure 1), it is now accepted that setting out principles or guidelines is insufficient without an effective

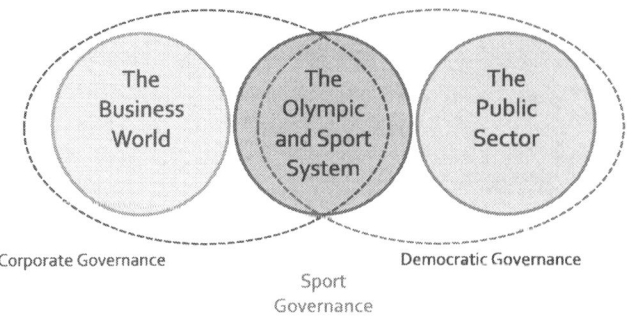

Figure 1. Sport governance at the intersection of corporate and democratic governances (after Henry and Lee 2004).

method for evaluating the governance of individual sport organizations. The first true set of governance indicators was the Basic Indicators for Better Governance of International Sport (BIBGIS), published by Chappelet and Mrkonjic in 2013, although the IOC's 'Basic Universal Principles of good governance of the Olympic and sports movement' (IOC 2008) could be considered a governance checklist. Known as the BUPs, this long catalogue of some 120 guidelines (mostly expressed as recommendations) was drawn up in 2008 and approved by the Olympic Congress in 2009. In contrast, the BIBGIS consists of 63 indicators covering seven areas of governance: Organisational transparency, Reporting transparency, Stakeholders' representation, Democratic process, Control mechanisms, Sport integrity and Solidarity. In 2015, the Danish organization Play the Game published its Sports Governance Observer, which uses 36 indicators to assess four areas of governance (Geeraert 2015). Also in 2015, the Australian government introduced 20 mandatory principles for sports governance (AIS 2015) and Sport England began promoting its Governance Strategy (SE, n.d.). National governing bodies in both these countries have to implement these guidelines in order to continue receiving government subsidies. At the end of the same year, the UK government's strategy for sport (HMG 2015) called for a new governance code in the UK (section 8.4, pages 64, 65). In May of the following year, Britain's prime minister, David Cameron, hosted an anti-corruption summit in London. His wish that the summit also address sport resulted in the two government agencies responsible for elite and grassroots sport publishing a Charter for Sports Governance (UK Sport & Sport England 2016). In fact, this charter is merely a precursor to a new code of governance for sport organizations, which is due to come into effect in 2017 but which was not ready for publication at the time of the summit.

Finally, in 2016, the General Assembly of the Association of Summer Olympic International Federations (ASOIF) endorsed 50 governance indicators covering five key principles (ten indicators for each principle: Transparency, Integrity, Democracy, Sports development and solidarity, and Control mechanisms), drawn up by an ad hoc taskforce (ASOIF 2016). The IFs within the ASOIF must now assess whether these indicators are respected in their organization. These audits will be in addition to the financial audits required under Swiss law (article 69b of Switzerland's Civil Code) for large IFs based in Switzerland. The IOC demanded the introduction of such a monitoring system as a way of ensuring the large sums it distributes to the IFs from Olympic Games revenues are used appropriately (IOC 2015). At the same time (IOC 2015), the IOC's Executive Board asked the Institute of Management Development (IMD), a business school based in Lausanne, to audit the IOC's governance.

Governance has to be monitored over time in order to determine whether it is improving. Rather than the 'good governance' so often alluded to since the World Bank first popularized the term, the objective should be to ensure 'better governance' within each organization. The focus should be on helping sport organizations improve, not on producing meaningless rankings based on comparisons between very different, and therefore fundamentally incomparable, sport organizations.

Monitoring of sports governance

Carrying out such regular monitoring, which focuses mainly on internal operations, is not always easy, as is shown by the difficulties encountered by FIFA's Audit and Compliance Committee (ACC). In fact, concerns over his independence led the chair of the ACC to resign in May 2016 (Gibson 2016) as he could be removed by a simple vote of the FIFA Council.

Four scenarios can be envisaged for carrying out this monitoring. The first scenario is for each sport organization to set up an internal entity to monitor its entire range of activities (not just its finances, although this is central). This is what the World Bank did when it created the World Bank Inspection Panel (WBIP), which assesses all the projects the Bank finances, some of which have been accused of corruption and of not promoting sustainable development. Such auditing entities must be independent and linked to the host organization's governing body, which must appoint members either permanently or on long-term mandates. Recent reforms within FIFA included the creation of such an entity, named the Audit and Compliance Committee, a step the body responsible for overseeing FIFA's reform process, the Independent Governance Committee, considered essential (See Scala's chapter in Pieth 2014). In 2007, The IAAF, as part of its governance reforms, created the Athletics Integrity Board and Unit to support its work in the field of integrity, including doping but also corruption, match-fixing, etc. This 4-member Board is elected by the IAAF Congress (of national associations = IAAF members) and reporting to it on a regular basis

The second scenario is to entrust monitoring to outside specialists, for example, one of the 'big four' accounting firms. In Switzerland, appointing external auditors has been obligatory since 2005 for nonprofit associations (most international sport organizations are associations) that exceed two of three thresholds set by Swiss law (article 69b of the Civil Code): turnover of more than CHF20 million; assets of more than CHF10 million; more than 50 employees. Such an audit should go beyond financial aspects and be totally independent, which is difficult to achieve because the auditor receives its remuneration from the organization it is auditing. For example, questions are still being asked about the absence of warnings from FIFA's external auditors prior to 2015 (KPMG) or, perhaps, the failure to act on these warnings. In fact, KPMG resigned as FIFA auditors in 2016 because of the potential systemic risk to its reputation.

The third scenario is to create a specialist body to monitor and help improve the governance of all international sport organizations. The World Anti-Doping Agency (WADA), set up in 1999 to coordinate the global fight against doping, could provide a model for such a body. In fact, many people continue to call for the creation of a World Anti-Corruption Agency (WACA) or for a less constraining International Sport Integrity Partnership (ISIP).

Because creating this type of monitoring or surveillance organization or scheme would undoubtedly generate resistance and apprehension, it would probably be necessary to conclude an international convention (as was done for WADA) to ensure public authorities across the globe cooperate in the fight to eliminate what can be termed 'the dark side of sport'. Switzerland, as the main host of international sport organizations, could sponsor such a convention. Another long-standing example of cooperation in the world of international sport is provided by the Court of Arbitration for Sport (CAS), which was set up in 1983 under Swiss law and whose authority is now accepted by all Olympic sport organizations, including FIFA (last IF to accept).

The fourth scenario is a sort of compromise between the second and third scenarios. It is inspired by the audits of intergovernmental organizations within the UN, which involve appointing auditors on the basis of regular calls for tenders from specialist national auditing bodies known for their independence and impartiality. For example, in recent years the World Intellectual Property Organization (WIPO) has been audited by Switzerland's Federal Audit Office, which, in this case, reports to the member states that form WIPO's governing body (and to the public via WIPO's website). Hence, member states receive assessments and recommendations that do not originate from the organization's management or a private service provider whose conclusions may not be entirely impartial.

All of these scenarios involve costs, but they could also generate savings and synergies for sport organizations if they could pool their efforts as they do in anti-doping with the Sport-Accord dedicated unit. They can be implemented in parallel and on a voluntary basis, which would facilitate their adoption. However, one thing is clear: the status quo has become untenable and, given the damage done to the reputation of international sport in 2015 and 2016, a solution must be found very quickly.

In addition, there are three important questions relating to sports governance that have almost never been addressed. The first is the use of funds distributed to the members of IFs (national federations) or Olympic stakeholders (mostly IFs and National Olympic Committees – NOCs). Are these funds being used 'correctly' in order to develop sport? Is there not a risk they may end up in the pockets of local sports administrators? To mitigate this risk, the IOC's NOCs Relations Department has developed a self-assessment tool called UMAP (Understanding, Managing, Auditing, Planning), which is available online to all NOCs around the world.

The second question concerns the fact that, in nearly all sport organizations, the president is responsible for running both the organization's regulation activities (under the board's control) and its business activities. This trend was started by Samaranch, when he became president of the IOC in 1980 (Chappelet 2014), and by Blatter, when he was elected president of FIFA in 1998. In other words, in most sport organizations, the CEO is also the chairman of the board, a state of affairs that is frowned upon by many corporate governance guidelines (see, for example, The UK Corporate Governance Code, June 2010, section A.3.1), even though this issue remains open to debate in the literature (e.g. Tonello 2011). A candidate to the FIFA presidency in 2016 proposed that the roles of regulation and commercialization be clearly separated by creating two different organisations in charge of each roles, but he was not elected.

The third question arises from the way host cities (or, in some cases, countries or national federations) for major sports events are chosen. The attribution of major events has generated numerous scandals that have led to governance reforms (selection of Salt Lake City to host the 2002 Winter Olympics, selection of Qatar for the 2022 Football World Cup, selection of host cities for the World Championships in Athletics, etc.). Depending on the statutes of the organizations in question, host cities tend to be chosen by a small number of electors (around 100 at the IOC, 200 at FIFA, 20 at the IAAF), which makes the system more susceptible to corruption. One solution would be to greatly increase the number of electors by expanding electorates to include, for example, former Olympians (athletes who have taken part in the Olympics), former players in the World Cup, athletes or fans, etc. Such a massive increase in the number of voters would substantially reduce the risk of corruption. No organization has, as yet, contemplated such a reform, as it would have to be approved by the very people who currently choose host cities/nations/federations and who would thereby lose some of their power. But such a reform could be adopted for future decisions, thereby delaying the loss of power and the resistance of current voters. FIFA's response, as part of its 2015 governance reforms, was to transfer this electoral power from its executive committee (25 members) to the FIFA Congress (209 members in 2015), which, unsurprisingly, was happy to approve a reform that gave it more power.

A useful model of governance

Pérez's (2003) model for corporate governance provides a useful template for analysing sports governance because it differentiates between five levels of governance, from day-to-day management to the legal framework governing an organization's operations. This model (Figure 2) was designed to address five fundamental questions concerning corporate governance. Although it was drawn up for the business sector, it can also be applied to sport organizations.

Applying this model to the IOC produces the following pyramid (see Figure 3), following the reforms introduced in 1999 in the wake of the Salt Lake City scandal (for more details, see Chappelet 2012).

The first three levels of Pérez's model depend mostly on internal structures and statutes set up by the organization in question. In contrast, the top two levels (4 and 5) require government supervision via national or international law.

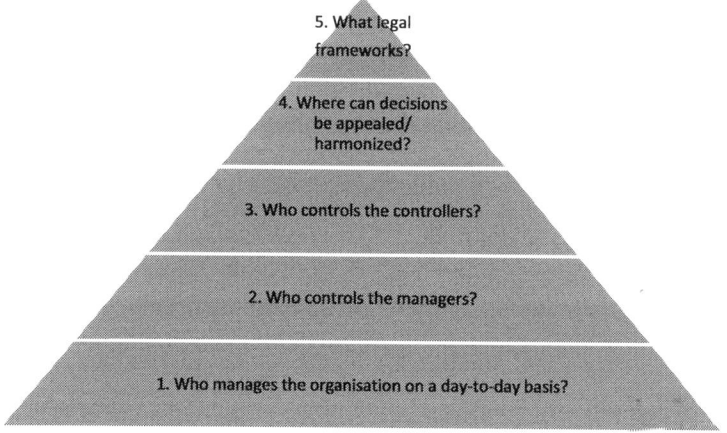

Figure 2. The five questions associated with Pérez's five levels of governance.

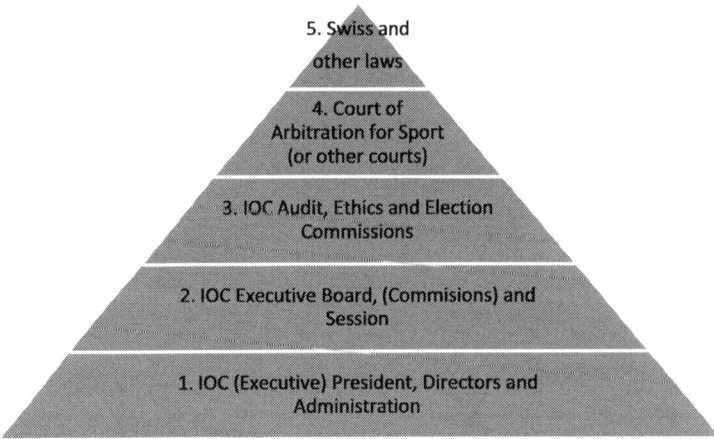

Figure 3. Pérez's model applied to the IOC.

The IOC falls mostly under the jurisdiction of Swiss law because, like many other international sport organizations, it is based in Switzerland and subject to articles 60–79 of the Swiss civil code (for Swiss nonprofit associations). It is also subject to other Swiss laws and to the Court of Arbitration for Sport (set up under chapter 12 of the Swiss federal law on international private law), which is recognized by all the IFs of Olympic sports as the supreme body for settling sport related disputes. Olympic sports organizations accept the need to collaborate with national governments, as long as they retain their autonomy. The 'price' they pay for this autonomy is an obligation to implement 'good governance' (see, for example, point 7 of the BUPs: 'Harmonious relations with governments while preserving autonomy', IOC 2008).

Currently, there is little international legislation that can be directly applied to sport. The exceptions to this rule fall into four areas and are covered by four international treaties/ conventions:

- Sports events spectator violence (Council of Europe 1985), integrated safety (Council of Europe 2016).
- Doping (UNESCO 2005).
- Match-fixing (Council of Europe 2014).
- (Public and private) corruption (United Nations 2003).

However, there is an increasing tendency for governments that have ratified these treaties to draw up or amend national laws in order to cover sport. For example, changes to Swiss law have led to a number of prosecutions in the country's civil courts (FIFA, doping and other affairs, see Chappelet 2010). Investigations have also been carried out by prosecutors in countries hosting sports events and French prosecutors have looked into the affairs of the IAAF (the accused IAAF president was resident in France). In 2016, Brazil's justice department brought charges in a case of ticket-touting involving an IOC member and a Brazilian court ordered the seizure of Olympic Broadcast Services' assets after the company was accused of breaking labour laws at the 2016 Olympic Games in Rio de Janeiro.

Most significantly, US law is playing an ever more important role in international sport. For example, it was the US Department of Justice that ordered the arrest of a dozen FIFA executives in Switzerland and, in 2016, the US attorney's office for the Eastern District of New York started investigating allegations of doping at the 2014 Winter Olympics in Sochi, Russia. American prosecutors are able to do this thanks to the Racketeer Influenced and Corrupt Organization (RICO) Act, which extends their jurisdiction well beyond the United States under certain circumstances (Henning 2016).

Improving the regulation of international sport: a possible solution

The growth of sport during the twentieth century led to misconduct in areas other than spectator violence (hooliganism), doping and match-fixing, which, as noted in the previous section, are subject to international conventions and, once these conventions have been ratified, to provisions of national laws passed thereafter. Although many forms of financial corruption are covered by the anti-corruption conventions drawn up by organizations such as the United Nations, Council of Europe and Organization for Economic Cooperation and Development, corruption in (private) sport organizations can take many non-financial forms, including using inducements to influence the attribution of sports events, the trafficking of children and the violation of workers' rights, etc. All of these issues affect the integrity of sport and damage the credibility sport needs in order to generate revenues through ticket sales, sponsorship and broadcasting rights (Pound 2016).

Several authors have suggested ways of combating these problems and thereby improving the regulation of international sport. In 2014, the IOC created an internal Ethics and Compliance Office (in addition to its Ethics Commission, set up in 1999). Chappelet (2011) argued for the creation of an Olympic accountability watchdog, and the World Anti-Doping Agency used the 2011 European Union Sports Forum to call for the creation of a global anti-corruption agency (Harris 2011). Launched in April 2016 under the auspices of the International Centre for Sport Security (ICSS 2016), the Sport Integrity Global Alliance (SIGA) has published its Universal Standards of Sport Integrity (October 2016). Also in 2016, the IOC set up a Joint Integrity Intelligence Unit in order to monitor and assess any potential unethical activities at the Rio Olympics, as was done with respect to match-fixing for London 2012 (Chappelet 2015). Three British and Irish boxers were reprimanded for betting on the Rio 2016 boxing competitions, even though they were not participating (Ingle 2016). Finally, in February 2016, the IOC launched its International Sports Integrity Partnership (ISIP) at a major conference in Lausanne.

Although these initiatives have their value, they have not managed to involve the world's national governments, without which levels 4 and 5 of Pérez's governance model cannot be implemented. A more effective solution than voluntary 'alliances' or 'partnerships' would be to adopt an international convention linking national governments and sports organizations in the same way that the Geneva Conventions bring together signatory states and the governmental and non-governmental bodies that make up the International Red Cross and Red Crescent Movement (IRCRCM).

These Conventions were drafted in 1949 on the basis of the 1864 Geneva Convention, signed when the International Committee of the Red Cross was formed, have now been ratified by 188 countries (against 183 countries for the UNESCO anti-doping convention in 2016). They lay out the framework within which the IRCRCM operates and cover the humanitarian rights of soldiers wounded during wars, shipwreck victims, prisoners of war and civilians in enemy-controlled territory.

One or more conventions (which could be known as the 'Lausanne Conventions' in honour of the role this city has played in the development of international sport) could be drawn up to provide an international legal framework, in the sense of Pérez's model (2003), for world sport that would combat the 'dark side of sport' and promote its 'bright side'. Such a Lausanne convention could create a body to audit sports organizations, as discussed in the second part of this article.

Conclusion

Adequate sports governance cannot exist without greater government involvement in regulating international sport and, consequently, national sport. Only governments can provide a national legal framework (fifth and final level of Pérez's model of governance) and prepare the ground for drawing up a treaty or convention as the basis for international sports legislation. Such a treaty is becoming increasingly indispensable for a global sector with many cases of misconduct in several areas, including doping, match-fixing, hooliganism, racism, human rights violations and corruption. This regulation must respect the autonomy of sport organizations, as recommended by the Council of Europe's European Sports Charter. In terms of the integrity of sport, guaranteeing the 'responsible autonomy' of sport organizations, most of which are nonprofit organizations, in exchange for adequate governance is arguably the best compromise between state and private control.

The alternative of state control is not realistic in so far as national governments have other priorities than sporting activities and performance (which would, in that case, be managed by public bodies rather than nonprofit associations) and do not have the means to finance sports activities (which are currently self-financed by the revenues from major sporting events, most notably the Olympic Games). The privatization of activities linked to sporting performance could be envisaged, as is the case for several sports in North America, but this would quickly turn sport into a branch of the entertainment industry. In fact, the United States' major professional leagues (MLB, NBA, MLS and, more recently, NFL) are for-profit corporations subject to taxation. Following a proposal put forward by an MP from Zurich named Cédric Wermuth (2016), Switzerland's parliament could soon debate the issue of how major IFs are taxed and the possibility of changing their legal form.

Hence, sport organizations and their governance are destined to combine elements of corporate governance (from the private sector) with aspects of democratic governance (from the public sector), as shown in Figure 1. Only intergovernmental treaties can provide the international legal framework needed to oversee this new form of sport governance. Benefits and drawbacks of such a convention or conventions should be further studied.

Disclosure statement

No potential conflict of interest was reported by the author.

References

AFP. 2015. *FIFA and IAAF Scandals Warning for Corrupt Sports Administrators*, December 30. Accessed October 1, 2016. www.dawn.com/news/1229640

AIS. 2015. *Australian Mandatory Sports Governance Principles*, June. Australian Government, Australian Sports Commission. Accessed October 1, 2016. www.ausport.gov.au/supporting/ governance/mandatory_sports_governance_principles

ASOIF. 2016. *ASOIF Governance Task Force (GTF) – 1st Report to ASOIF Council*. Lausanne: Association of Summer Olympic International Federations.

Bevir, M. 2010. *Democratic Governance*. Princeton, NJ: University Press.

Chappelet, J.-L. 2010. *The Autonomy of Sport in Europe*. Strasbourg: Council of Europe Publishing.

Chappelet, J.-L. 2011. "Towards Better Olympic Accountability." *Sport in Society* 14 (3): 319–331. doi:10.1080/17430437.2011.557268

Chappelet, J.-L. 2012. "From Daily Management to High Politics: The Governance of the International Olympic Committee." In *The Handbook of International Sport Management*, edited by L. Robinson, and R. Palmer, 7–25. London: Routledge.

Chappelet, J.-L. 2014. "Une vie consacrée au sport: Juan Antonio Samaranch [A Life Dedicated to Sport: Juan Antonio Samaranch]." In *Les grands dirigeants du sport* [The Leaders of Sport], edited by E. Bayle, 237–252. Bruxelles: De Boeck.

Chappelet, J.-L. 2015. "The Olympic Fight against Match-fixing." *Sport in Society* 18 (10): 1260–1272. doi:10.1080/17430437.2015.1034519

Chappelet, J.-L., and M. Mrkonjic. 2013. *Basic Indicators for Better Governance in International Sport (BIBGIS): An Assessment Tool for International Sport Governing Bodies*. Lausanne: IDHEAP Working Paper, 1/2013.

Council of Europe. 1985. *European Convention on Spectator Violence and Misbehaviour at Sports Events and in Particular at Football Matches*, August. Strasbourg: Council of Europe.

Council of Europe. 2014. *Convention on the Manipulation of Sports Competition*, September. Macolin: Council of Europe. This Convention was Totally Revised in 2016.

Council of Europe. 2016. *Convention on an Integrated Safety, Security and Service Approach at Football Matches and Other Sports Events*, July. Strasbourg: Council of Europe.

EOC. 2001. *Statement of Good Governance Principles, "The Rules of the Game" First International Governance in Sport Conference*, January. Brussels.

EU. 2000. *Nice Declaration on the Specific Characteristics of Sport and Its Social Function in Europe, Adopted by the European Council in Nice*.

EU. 2013. *Principles of Good Governance in Sport*, September. Deliverable 2, Brussels: Expert Group "Good Governance".

Geeraert, A. 2015. *Sports Governance Observer 2015: The Legitimacy Crisis in International Sports Governance*. Copenhagen: Play The Game.

Gibson, O. 2016. "Fifa's Independent Audit Committee Chairman Resigns in Protest at Reforms." *The Guardian*, May 14.

Harris, N. 2011. "Head of WADA Calls for Global Anti-corruption Body." *Sporting Intelligence*, February 23. www.sportingintelligence.com/2011/02/23/head-of-wada-calls-for-global-anti-corruption-body-230201.

Henning, P. J. 2016. "Road Map for Pursuit of Soccer Charges." *International New York Times*, June 29, 14.

Henry, I., and P. C. Lee. 2004. "Governance and Ethics in Sport." In *The Business of Sport Management*, edited by J. Beech and S. Chadwick, 25–42. Harlow: Prentice Hall.

HMG. 2015. *Sporting Future: A New Strategy for an Active Nation*, December. London: Her Majesty's Government.

ICSS. 2016. *New Sport Integrity Global Alliance (SIGA) Launched*, April. Madrid. Accessed October 1, 2016. www.theicss.org/en/news/read/new-sport-integrity-global-alliance-siga-launched

Ingle, S. 2016. "IOC Reprimands British and Irish Boxers for Betting on Rio Olympics Bouts." *The Guardian*, September 28.

IOC. 2008. *Basic Universal Principles of Good Governance of the Olympic and Sports Movement*. Lausanne: International Olympic Committee.

IOC. 2015. *IOC Executive Board Adopts Declaration on Good Governance in Sport and the Protection of Clean Athletes*, Press Release, 15 December. Accessed October 1, 2015. www.olympic.org/news/ioc-executive-board-adopts-declaration-on-good-governance-in-sport-and-the-protection-of-clean-athletes

Mallin, C. A. 2011. *Handbook on International Corporate Governance: Country Analyses*. 2nd ed. Cheltenham: Edward Elgar.

Pérez, R. 2003. *La gouvernance de l'entreprise* [Corporate Governance]. Paris: la découverte.

Pieth, M., ed. 2014. *Reforming FIFA*. Zurich: Dike Verlag.

Pound, R. 2016. "If Football Doesn't Get a Grip, Fans Will Turn off the Money Tap." *The Telegraph*, September 30.

SE. n.d. *Sport England Sport Governance Strategy: On Board for Better Governance*. London: Sport England.

Tonello, M. 2011. "Separation of Chair and CEO Roles." *Harvard Law School Forum on Corporate Governance and Financial Regulation*, September 1, Accessed October 1, 2016. https://corpgov. law.harvard.edu/2011/09/01/separation-of-chair-and-ceo-roles/#2b

UK Sport & Sport England. 2016. *A Charter for Sports Governance in the United Kingdom*. London: UK Sport & Sport England.

UNESCO. 2005. *International Convention against Doping in Sport*, October. Paris: United Nations Education, Science and Culture Organisation.

United Nations. 2003. *Convention against Corruption*, October. New York: United Nations.

Wenn, S., R. Barney, and S. Martyn. 2011. *Tarnished Rings: The International Olympic Committee and the Salt Lake City Bid Scandal*. Syracuse: Syracuse University Press.

Wermuth, C. 2016. *Fédérations sportives internationales. Conséquences d'un changement de la forme juridique* [International Sports Federations: Consequences of a Change of Legal Form]. MP Intervention of 16.06.2016.

Sport and politics in a complex age

David Hassan

ABSTRACT

This article examines the complex nature of the relationship between international sport and politics in the twenty-first century. It does so by considering the cultural and geo-political profiles of those countries that are expressly pursuing the hosting of major international sporting events, such as the Olympic Games and the FIFA World Cup. It focuses, on the emergence of a raft of 'new' countries seeking to stage such global mega-events and considers why they would be so keen to do so when, based on participation levels amongst their indigenous peoples such a decision would appear to have little popular support. More to the point, there would seem to be increasing commonality amongst these 'new' nation-states in terms of their political profiles, their attitudes towards minorities, their approach to the advancement of a rights agenda, and to their motivations for hosting major sporting events in the first instance. Ultimately the article poses the question of whether sport should readily lend its remaining credibility to such nation-states or whether its ready acquiescence of the same actually says more about its virtual preoccupation with commercial return, persistent mal-governance or, in some cases, corruption.

Introduction

It would be nice to think that politics has no place in sport. Yet were this the case many of the positive consequences of this relationship would be lost. Certainly, from the beginning of international competition in the late 1920s sport has been central to diplomatic relations between countries, such as those that existed between USA and China in the late 1960s, where suspicion and hostility had predominated. It has often been a unifying force too in divided societies, including in Northern Ireland, and generated patriotism that has assisted fledging political administrations achieve popular support. It also played an important role in the fall of Apartheid in South Africa and remains a key aspect of a range of development programmes in the Global South to this day (Black and Peacock 2013).

More to the point, in certain situations sport has been the *only* arena to convey political messages. Through the embodied resistance of sportspersons like Muhammed Ali, John Carlos and Tommie Smith, and Andy Flower and Henry Olonga powerful, if uncomfortable messages for those in authority, have been played out (Hargreaves 2000). In the field of gender politics too, as sport is too often the site for the construction and reconstruction of hegemonic masculinity in society, women, including the Williams sisters in tennis, Katie Taylor in boxing and Tanya Gray Thompson in para-athletics have all challenged out-dated stereotypes that traditionally may have constrained participation or prevented it altogether (Adams 2016; Hargreaves 2000).

Yet, it is undoubtedly in the act of hosting major sporting events that the most potent political messages are formed (Horne 2016). For some countries this again can be a powerful, indeed liberating, experience. The hosting of the 1995 Rugby World Cup by South Africa, shortly after the end of the Apartheid era, conveyed a symbolism that few other mediums could have achieved as readily (Preuss 2007). Similarly the Summer Olympic Games of 2000, staged in Sydney, created a context in which the State could finally, and publically, express its profound regret concerning the treatment of Australia's Aboriginal community, in particular those affected by the so-called 'lost generation'. This was demonstrated in the response of the Australian nation to the medal winning performances of Cathy Freeman and how her successes clearly resonated beyond the athletics arena into all aspects of civic and political society (Hargreaves 2000).

It's true also however that major sporting events, notably the 1936 Berlin Olympics and the Summer Games staged in Munich in 1972, have been examples of the exploitation of sport for purely political ends. The 1936 Games, designed to showcase the strength of Nazi Germany, are regarded as the *bête noir* of the Olympic movement, even if the achievement of the American track athlete Jesse Owens served to somewhat undermine this claim (Horne and Whannel 2016). Similarly, the deaths of 11 Israeli athletes in 1972 ahead of the Munich games poignantly illustrated that, very often, sport can prove disproportionately impactful for those seeking to convey a political agenda, precisely because it is thought to be above the political realm. It's, therefore, around the broader significance of hosting major sporting events that the author wishes to make some comment and consider, in particular, what the future of this relationship may turn out to be. It is precisely because the very act of hosting an international sporting event conveys a range of desirable messages, both explicitly and implicitly understood, that it appears the desire to do so has never been greater (Preuss 2007).

Indeed, the past decade has represented an unprecedented period of development within world sport. A host of global events, everything from the Olympic Games to a range of World Championships, have been awarded to countries of modest international standing, certainly in sporting terms. This may be welcomed as the further globalization of this industry through the uncovering of new markets, as many of these countries are hosting events for the very first time. Yet closer scrutiny of these emerging nations reveals commonalities that may prove significant in the future direction of global sport. As such, on the one side of this equation sit a collection of 'new' nation-states who regard sport as a credible, even necessary, investment towards realizing their aim of full global emancipation. On the other exists an ever more complex sports governance network defined, in this era of neo-liberalism, by a pursuit of these very same 'new markets' amid the effective and expeditious 'privatisation' of world sport.

The challenge therefore is to consider why these 'new lands', to borrow a phrase used by the former FIFA President Sepp Blatter, are drawn to sport. For many of the Gulf States, such as Bahrain, UAE and Qatar, and others including Belarus, Equatorial Guinea, Uganda and Azerbaijan could, with the greatest of respect to them, never be described as leading nations in sporting terms yet between them, they either have already or will in the coming years, host almost every major global sporting tournament. Qatar alone staged more than 40 major international sporting events during 2015, yet is barely the size of a modest county in Great Britain either in terms of land mass or population (Kilgallen 2013). All of this would be sufficient to provoke some consideration of their motivations yet these countries, alongside others like Russia, China and Kazakhstan, share a common system of political organization, which is best described as authoritarian. As such it's not entirely clear how the greater acquiescence of sport by countries operating under this particular form of political regimes will play out in the future. In addition, there is a danger that the increasingly unregulated manner of awarding major sporting events to host nations may give rise to unintended consequences of a political nature (Hoye and Cuskelly 2007).

Theoretical context

Ultimately, therefore, it is necessary to consider whether, (a) The appropriation of sport by these countries assists their further maturity, as many are only recently established in international terms; (b) Whether the often lavish staging of these sporting events is designed to act as a form of cultural resistance against established 'Western' principles and practices; and/or (c) even that this considerable momentum on the hosting of major events provokes a realignment of any 'core'/'periphery' relationships that may persist between these nation-states and others.

In keeping with the work of Walt Rostow, international sport assists a nation's so-called 'drive to maturity', an era defined by social and economic prosperity (Rostow 1990). Yet, this maturation process is not an even one and whilst some countries may retain enviable levels of Gross Domestic Profit (GDP) with seemingly uninhibited access to natural resources, socially, culturally and, indeed, politically they may remain in the early stages of their development. Thus, for an ideal state of maturity to be achieved societies must present as 'fully developed' and thus, the hosting of major sporting events serves, at least in part, to convey this message (Rostow 1990). Yet, there remains a constant state of flux between the concept of 'modernisation', an essentially Western, normative term, and the 'traditional' and many emerging States continue to struggle with this juxtaposition. It is possible, for instance, to observe the 'hyper-modernity' existing alongside the 'traditional' within otherwise advanced and highly developed cities such as Dubai and Doha in the Middle East (Kilgallen 2013).

In contrast, the Italian neo-Marxist Antonio Gramsci suggests that the real power within and between countries exists in the realm of culture, of which sport is a dominant element (Gramsci 1992). According to this perspective, it is possible to argue that for countries like Russia, China and certain former Eastern bloc countries, the hosting of major sporting events even constitutes an act of resistance against the 'West' – a counter-hegemonic process, to use Gramsci's terminology (Gramsci 1992). Using sport as a tool in this expressive struggle, for instance by hosting the most expensive Summer and Winter Games in modern Olympic history, previously marginalized States in international relations, like China and Russia, are able to reshape many of the latent messages surrounding them through sport. In essence they are effectively seeking to reinterpret their global positioning by embracing the ethical value of elite competition and endeavour and its associated values (Black and Peacock 2013).

Yet, all of this runs the risk of somehow under-playing the commercial and economic reality of modern sport. Sport is an important generator of economic investment – the transformation of Barcelona as a major commercial European city following its hosting of the Summer Olympic Games in 1992, being a perfect case in point (Preuss 2007). In this respect, Wallerstein's work in the field of 'World Systems Analysis' reflects a classic materialist epistemology (Wallerstein 2004). This is one in which the core consists of Western so-called 'strong' states, with an internationally commercially active elite that concentrates wealth, and a comparatively, 'weak' or under-developed periphery too often exploited by the core. On Wallerstein's account, the core seeks to extend its profitability, which redefines the concept of 'international' as 'hegemonic', to under-developed markets. Of course this approach is often criticized precisely for its economic and political determinism, as it downplays the capacity of the so-called 'exploited' to retain some degree of self-determinism, not least in economic terms (Wallerstein 2004).

Whilst historically the majority of the World's leading sports events have been hosted in western liberal democracies, mostly European nation-states – for example, of the 55 Summer or Winter Olympics that have taken place in the modern Olympic era, two in every three have been staged in Europe (a figure incidentally that rises to four in every five if one other country, the USA, is included) this allowed for a cultural and in particular economic superiority to be exercised across much of the remainder of the world, and thereby create a peripheral reliance on established 'western' systems and practices in the presentation of global sport that went largely unquestioned (Horne and Whannel 2016). However, as previously semi-peripheral and peripheral states, in fact States that weren't even established or certainly that remained largely unknown, have sought a greater share of international sporting equity, this historical system, certainly in the realm of sport, of peripheral subjugation has begun to wither, albeit unevenly. The emergence of a raft of 'new' countries has significantly weakened the established global sporting order and whilst still some way short of Wallerstein's predicted 'systemic crisis' has cast an uneven and uncertain future for world sport (Wallerstein 2004).

Yet a disconnection between the practices, norms and values of the 'core' and those of the 'periphery' in State-sponsored sport persists and is most apparent, as suggested, in their internal political organization. Many of these 'new' nation-states are still on a pathway to full democracy, if that is their wish, and are ruled instead by a system of governance that is either totalitarian, monarchist or where power is retained centrally. Alongside latent concerns regarding the protection of other forms of freedom of expression this has left many traditional, established liberal democracies increasingly exasperated, if perhaps no less inclined to engage in a bidding war for major sporting tournaments evermore uncertain about the terms of engagement. An example of this was the 2015 decision by the Oslo Organizing Committee to withdraw its aspiration of hosting the 2022 Winter Olympics, when faced with rival bids from Kazakhstan and China. Interestingly, this decision was announced following a vote in the Norwegian parliament, which mirrored similar votes taken in Munich and St Moritz, which arrived at a similar decision to withdraw interest in hosting events that began, financially speaking, to take on a life of their own (Horne and Whannel 2016).

Whilst such objectives are externally focussed, what if anything, does the hosting of major events achieve for the population of these countries? It appears that sport in this guise is not about 'speaking' to the indigenous people of a country. Whereas the political scientist Ernest

Gellner argues persuasively that a sense of nationalism emerges only when States become recognizably formed and begin maturing, during the era of modernity, there is little sign of this process in many of the peripheral States now drawn to sport. The FIFA World Cup in Qatar, for example, is not about establishing a coherent sense of national identity for the Qatari people; neither is the 2017 IAAF World Cross Country Championships in Uganda about internal reform of its political systems (Gellner 1998; Horne 2016).

Governance

All of this brings to the fore the question of effective management of global sport (Hoye and Cuskelly 2007). The self-governed hierarchic networks that have traditionally existed in the sports world are increasingly facing attempts by governments and other empowered stakeholder organizations to interfere in their policy- and decision-making processes, and often, it might be argued, for good reason. The 2015 decision to award the 2021 IAAF World Championships to Eugene, Oregon was noteworthy on two counts. Firstly, Gothenburg believed itself to be actively engaged in a rival bid for the 2021 event and was taken aback, to put it mildly, by a seemingly unilateral decision on the part of the IAAF to simply side for the USA bid. Secondly, Eugene, a city with a population barely in excess of 100,000 people, is also the home of the sportswear manufacturer Nike, which may have been a consideration in the final decision of the IAAF. Such developments reflect the emergence of a greater networked governance approach to sport to the detriment of the traditional form of self-governance, which was itself of course subject to increasing criticism from sports followers following a series of high-profile scandals and controversies (Hoye and Cuskelly 2007).

These concerns continue in the face of the then FIFA General Secretary Jerome Valcke's assertion, prior to the 2014 World Cup Finals, that 'less democracy is sometimes better for organising a World Cup' (Horne 2016, 34), which perhaps explains why the next two tournaments will take place in Russia and Qatar. Remarkably, Bernie Ecclestone, the CEO of the Formula One Group that owns the broadcast rights for F1, gave an almost verbatim reprise of these comments at the recent Bahrain GP claiming that the sport had, in his eyes, become 'too democratic'. It appears, despite the perception of sport as having a natural home within established liberal democracies, that the future for high-level sport is in those settings where things happen unquestionably, whatever the price (Hoye and Cuskelly 2007).

In less than 10 years, the Arab world has emerged as a dominant player in world sport (Kilgallen 2013; O'Connor 2013). How better to illustrate your advances as a modern nation than to host major sporting tournaments, to do so lavishly and to remain part of public discourse for many years in advance of a World Cup or Olympic Games. Sport, to parallel the work of Rostow (1990), is clearly a key component of any maturation strategy employed by GCC States. Yet, it's also the case that many of the Gulf States retain an uncompromising attitude towards dissenters and are viewed by some as repressive in their approach towards women in particular, which begins to make problematic sport's ready acquiescence of these same nation-states. There really is a danger that the wrong messages are sent out to observers about where the moral and ethical compass of sport, in its most generic of forms, is pointing (Forsythe 2009).

Previously, in 2008, China's first ever Olympic Games paralleled the country's emergence as a global economic power and showcased a political order whose rigidity and sense of discipline supposedly produced results. Whilst on so many fronts and for some considerable period of time, China existed on the periphery of international relations, its hosting of the Summer Games conveyed an almost ineffable sense of legitimacy that redefined its marginal status (Horne and Whannel 2016). Yet, it is this uncomfortable relationship between the use of sport to confirm a move to a fully inclusive China and the reality of a country that continues to justify punitive acts in order to preserve 'social stability' that represents continued cause for concern. Yet, more than ever, not least on account of its remarkable investment into sports like association football, is would appear the future of sport is to be found in the Far East and China in particular, as the epicentre of sport moves evermore decisively from its traditional setting of Europe (Riordan and Jones 1999).

During the 33-year rule of President Mbasogo Equatorial Guinea has regularly been included in Freedom House's list of the world's most repressive regimes. The country, known for its lamentable levels of corruption, neglect of widespread poverty, and an uncompromising criminal justice system, was selected as one of the hosts of the Africa Cup of Nations in 2015. Notwithstanding the context in which this decision was served, coming as it did in the wake of an Ebola outbreak on the continent of Africa, it risks conveying entirely the wrong messages to a watching international audience about the ethical context in which sport takes place.

Similarly, in 2014, the decision by the International Ice Hockey Federation to stage its World Championships in Belarus represented the source of some regret for followers of the sport, in particular. Under the rule of Alyaksandr Lukashenka, once dubbed the last dictator in Europe, Belarus is best known for its unethical electoral systems, the rendition of outspoken opponents, and the world's longest lists of political prisoners.

In the Summer of 2015, Azerbaijan hosted the first ever European Olympics, despite ranking 156th out of 179 in the Reporters Without Borders world press freedom index and described by Amnesty as 'a template lesson in how to launder a country's image through sport'. Despite these concerns, the country's capital Baku, also staged an F1 race in 2016 and will host group games during the European football Championships of 2020. Commenting on the F1 race planned for Baku, Bernie Ecclestone said (there) 'doesn't seem to be any big problem (with human rights)' despite at least 33 human rights protestors, journalists and opposition politicians being detained without trial in the country in 2015 alone. Again there is a sense in which the extraordinary price paid for sporting events can be justified as part of a wider strategy towards a globally recognized maturity (Horne 2016).

Hosts of both the recent 2014 Sochi Winter Games and the 2018 World Cup finals, Russia is staging more international tournaments over the next five years than any other nation in the world, despite continued controversy over its relationship with Ukraine and similar international concerns. Its lavish spending on the recent Winter Olympics staged in Sochi in 2014, three times more than spent on the Summer Olympics held in London during August 2012, was a flexing of economic power unparalleled in modern sport, a counter-hegemonic act of the most powerful form. Of course Ukraine itself was the focus of considerable scrutiny during its co-hosting of the 2012 Euro Championships following the jailing of former Prime Minister Tymoshenko on charges that most felt were expressly political in form. Last year Amnesty demanded the International Olympic Committee take Russia's leadership to task over what it interpreted as a 'blatant violation of human rights' in the context of the 2014 Games. 'Its failure to admonish the authorities for their on-going harassment is a failure to live up to the very principles that form the core of the Olympic Charter' it claimed.

After being left with a choice between two cities – Beijing and Almaty in Kazakhstan – as host of the 2022 Winter Olympics, the IOC has now passed a raft of reforms designed to entice more democratic countries to bid for such Games. It constitutes a remarkable intervention into politics by a major sporting body.

The 2017 IAAF World Cross Country Championships will be staged in Kampala, the capital of Uganda. This again despite the country having an unenviable record in terms of its own self-governance, including the embezzlement of almost $13 million of international aid, which led to a host of countries, including Ireland, withdrawing their support for this otherwise impoverished state. The IAAF's decision to award the 2017 Championships to Uganda, not to mention the 2019 event to Qatar, might offer some insight into last month's unilateral move by the IAAF to award the 2021 event to Eugene, America's self-proclaimed 'track city'. Yet now, for the very first time, rights protections will be included in host city contracts seeking to stage the Olympic Games, even if no other major events. According to Human Rights Watch 'This reform should give teeth to the lofty Olympic language that sport can be "a force for good"'.

The reality remains of course that many of these peripheral States can facilitate a defining agent of globalization, capitalist economics. Thus, if modern sport is categorized by extraordinary financial investment then such nations are well placed to meet this challenge and consider it only a small premium to pay for the projection of national legitimacy, if not unity, and evermore crucial to their full maturity as sovereign States. Nowhere is this more apparent it seems than in the Middle East, in particular the countries of the GCC. Collectively, they have taken the use of sport for non-sporting outcomes to an unparalleled level (Kilgallen 2013).

Middle East

As such amongst the dominant countries in world sport at present are those based in the Middle East, in particular Bahrain, UAE and Qatar, though interestingly not the largest country in the region, Saudi Arabia (O'Connor 2013). Their combined populations equate to 12.7 million people, less than either the cities of London or Paris. Qatar, with a total population of 2.1 million, has less people living there than do so in Birmingham in the British midlands, whilst more people reside in Glasgow than in the entire Kingdom of Bahrain. Yet their wealth and investment power is phenomenal. The UAE alone has a GDP of $402.3 bn, whilst Qatar has a GDP that, at $203.2 bn, represents more than half that figure but is drawn from only 20% of the UAE's population. If one were to combine the GDP of Qatar, Bahrain and UAE, it would figure amongst the Top 20 countries in the world in terms of overall wealth, include Saudi Arabia and this moves into a global top 12 position (Kilgallen 2013).

Qatar accumulates sporting events in a manner unmatched by any nation-state in the history of modern sport (Kilgallen 2013). Between November 2014 and November 2015, Qatar will have hosted the world championships in squash, short course swimming, handball, boxing and para-athletes, to name but a few. Yet one could comfortably situate Qatar inside a small part of the United Kingdom, e.g. Northern Ireland, and still have 20% landmass to spare. Similarly the cities of Milan, Barcelona or London are larger in area landmass than Bahrain, which has hosted a round of the Formula 1 Grand Prix for almost a decade and also staged the Gulf Cup, the region's foremost football tournament, in 2013.

UAE, with a total population of 9.3 million people but, crucially, an indigenous populous of less than 1 million, has managed to self-define itself as a modern, progressive, even Westernized nation-state, yet is barely four decades in existence. By defining itself through the hosting of major events, it has skilfully used sports commonly associated with other parts of the world to achieve this status. Abu Dhabi, although something of a new arrival to global city marketing, is determined to eclipse Dubai's more immediate name recognition through its use of sport, which is heavily profiled in the 'Abu Dhabi 2030' vision. The remarkable investments of the ruling Mansoor family, underpinned by an oil reserve 10 times that of Dubai, will make for an interesting period ahead as the State seeks to grow its already very prominent role in world sport (O'Connor 2013).

After the cancellation of the Formula 1 race in Bahrain during 2011, on the foot of a popular uprising in the country by the majority Shia population, part of the so-called Arab spring, the government response was swift. Widespread arrests of protestors and the expulsion of many foreign media outlets, including the BBC, was commonplace. Yet the approach of the FIA, motorsport's world governing body, was remarkable, notably again in its attitude to press ahead with the race in the face of internal ethnic conflict. Article 1 of the FIA Statutes clearly states that 'The FIA shall refrain from manifesting racial, political or religious discrimination in the course of its activities and from taking any action in this respect' (FIA Statutes, accessed on 23 November 2016). Yet the FIA's stance on the Bahrain GP, both in 2012 and again 2013, was expressly pro-Government, acting in favour of a Sunni minority administration that had invested heavily in hosting the Formula 1 race and was determined that its staging would convey a sense of normality to a watching international audience (O'Connor 2013).

Indeed, the on-going geo-political tensions within the Middle East remain something of a concern for onlookers. These are best illustrated through the campaign of Jordan's Prince Ali Bin Al-Hussein's attempt to replace Sepp Blatter as FIFA President in early 2015. Despite not being favoured by his own Asian confederation, who perhaps unsurprisingly offered its backing to Blatter, Al-Hussein retained the unlikely support of a raft of other national federations. For example, he was nominated for the post by the English FA, despite the other two contenders for the position representing fellow-UEFA nations, and seconded by the United States Soccer Federation, which typically adopts a passive approach to the internal politics of FIFA. These unlikely of allies can only be explained, in the minds of some, in the context of wider political alliances existing and emerging in the Middle East. This overt intervention of politics into sport in the region does not play well with observers, concerned with the potential for divisions to foster between neighbouring States and spiral into all aspects of everyday life, including sport.

The degree of rivalry between a host of GCC countries and Qatar is similarly noteworthy (Kilgallen 2013; O'Connor 2013). The deaths of over 200 workers in the act of building stadia for the 2022 World Cup, the astronomical rise in the numbers of cardiac arrests being suffered by many more who survive, and the regular ignominy these men – mostly from the Indian sub-continent – are subjected to, including being forced to compete during later 2014 in a failed attempt by the Qatari's to set a world record for participation in the marathon, has become an international story. In the field of motorsport, which has a particular association with the Gulf, Qatar's capture of a round of the Formula 1 championship from 2016 onwards came at a considerable cost. It has now become the single most expensive round of the F1 championship in motorsport history as an objection from Bahrain to the running of an F1 event incensed the Qatari's to such an extent that they paid considerably more to stage the event than the second most lucrative round of F1. Finally, at the recent World Handball Championships in Doha, not alone did Qatar hire an entire team of foreign nationals to compete for the nation it even transported fans from Spain to support them, these were people whose contract mandated them to back Qatar even if it was competing against Spain. This phenomenon is not new, with army and police personnel regularly being recruited to watch sporting events, but it does point to a fundamental problem when the State vision fails to be matched by the reality of what is happening 'on the ground' and, as this gap grows, so too does the scepticism of those looking on from the sidelines.

Conclusion

Sport nowadays is not only about big business, but also global politics, strategic influence, social well-being and economic performance (Horne 2016). Whilst some commentators decry the emergence of something akin to a twenty-first century sporting arms race, the reality is that many countries have long since realized how powerful sport is and have set about exploiting it for all, it seems, than sporting outcomes.

The picture that has emerged during this article is one in which there has been a considerable dislocation of a well-established global sports industry by the emergence of States, previously with only a passing interest in sport, at precisely the same point as the growth of sport worldwide has sought greater commodification of the sporting product. Yet all of this would be fathomable, indeed welcomed, were it not for the common political systems, the approach towards marginalized populations and the issue of rights more generally, demonstrated within these very same countries.

As such it is a fact that more and more sports events are being hosted by authoritarian states, using them to convey legitimacy and strengthen the power and profile of their rulers. On the other side of this, whereas those that govern sport traditionally would have looked to Western democracies as their natural place to do business, now they increasingly look east, to certain countries where money, rather than necessarily freedom, holds sway (Horne and Whannel 2016).

Ultimately, therefore, those States involved in this process seek to redefine, or simply define, their international image by shrouding themselves in the cloak of sporting respectability. Sport understood as 'European', 'Modern' and 'Enlightened' remains desirable for certain emerging nations. Sport for others represents a 'Trojan horse' amid a wider pursuit of international legitimacy, and improved trade relations, in a new world order driven by global capitalism. Ultimately, international sport comes with its own messages – how to behave, how to think and how to interpret one's place in the world. In the absence of a concerted, or coherent, approach on the part of developed or core nations to engage with emerging or peripheral States in any sustained way, sports governing bodies remain critical in any process of emancipation.

Disclosure statement

No potential conflict of interest was reported by the author.

References

Adams, M. 2016. "Feminist Politics and Sport." In *Routledge Handbook of Sport and Politics*, edited by A. Bairner, J. Kelly, and J. Lee, 35–51. London: Routledge.

Black, D., and B. Peacock. 2013. "Sport and Diplomacy." In *The Oxford Handbook of Modern Diplomacy*, edited by A. Cooper, J. Heine, and R. Thakur, 12–27. London: Oxford Press.

FIA Statutes. Vol. 1. Accessed November 23, 2016. www.fia.com

Forsythe, D. 2009. *Encyclopedia of Human Rights*. Vol. 1. London: Oxford University Press.

Gellner, E. 1998. *Nationalism*. Phoenix, AZ: Phoenix.

Gramsci, A. 1992. *Prison Notebooks: Volume 1*. New York: Columbia University Press.

Hargreaves, J. 2000. *Heroines of Sport: The Politics of Difference and Identity*. London: Routledge.

Horne, J. 2016. "The Contemporary Politics of Sport Mega-events." In *Routledge Handbook of Sport and Politics*, edited by A. Bairner, J. Kelly, and J. Lee, 89–103. London: Routledge.

Horne, J., and G. Whannel. 2016. *Understanding the Olympics*. London: Routledge.

Hoye, C., and G. Cuskelly. 2007. *Sport Governance*. Amsterdam: Elsevier.

Kilgallen, C. 2013. "Developing Elite Sporting Talent in Qatar: The Aspire Academy for Sports Excellence." In *Sport Management in the Middle East: A Case Study Analysis*, edited by M. B. Sulayem, S. O'Connor, and D. Hassan, 173–192. London: Routledge.

O'Connor, S. 2013. "Sport Consumers in the Middle East." In *Sport Management in the Middle East: A Case Study Analysis*, edited by M. B. Sulayem, S. O'Connor, and D. Hassan, 65–86. London: Routledge.

Preuss, H., ed. 2007. *The Impact and Evaluation of Major Sporting Events*. London: Routledge.

Riordan, J., and R. Jones. 1999. *Sport and Physical Education in China*. London: E&FN Spon.

Rostow, W. 1990. *The Stages of Economic Growth: A Non-communist Agenda*. Cambridge: Cambridge University Press.

Wallerstein, I. 2004. *World-systems Analysis*. London: Duke University Press.

Sport mega-events, the 'non-West' and the ethics of event hosting

Suzanne Dowse and Thomas Fletcher

ABSTRACT

Events and sports events are perceived as having the potential to contribute to a number of benefits for the host country and its communities. The socio-political and economic environment of the host is an important consideration for both prospective hosts and event owners when allocating hosting rights. It is therefore, unsurprising that concerns have been raised over the relatively recent relocation of events to developing countries which, by their nature, frequently lack the economic, political and social stability of the traditional industrialized host. Developing nations are less affluent and arguably less prepared to deliver large scale sports events than developed nations. Therefore, this paper asks, 'are governing bodies, when equipped with this knowledge, ethically obliged to withhold hosting rights from developing countries?' The paper argues that denying sovereign States the right to make their own decisions would appear to compound the disadvantaged status of countries that mega-event hosting is perceived to address. The paper contends that event hosts – particularly those in the developing world – are potentially vulnerable to exploitation by the event owner.

Introduction

Events and sports events are perceived as having the potential to contribute to a number of benefits for the host country and its communities. Amongst other things these include: bringing lasting social and economic benefits, enhancing national identity and image, regeneration and place (re)development, as well as facilitating community cohesion and well-being (Sharpley and Stone 2011). However, mega sports events (MSE) in particular are also known for their darker side. For example, they are frequently associated with corruption, soaring economic costs, environmental degradation, securitization, gentrification, violence and human rights violations (Dashper, Fletcher, and McCullough 2014). More routinely, principally via media coverage, sports events remain a primary agonist in the (re)articulation of structural inequalities, along the lines of gender, sexuality, 'race' and ethnicity, social class, disability, and their intersections (Fletcher and Dashper 2013). Thus, according to Hayes and Karamichas (2012, 2) MSEs are not simply sporting or cultural phenomena:

They are also political and economic events, characterized by the generation and projection of symbolic meanings – most obviously over the nature of statehood, economic power and collective cultural identity – and by social conflict, especially over land use, and over the extent and contours of public spending commitments.

Without a doubt, MSEs have significant consequences for the host community. These consequences flow from the scale and complexity of the event, and the logistics of delivering what is effectively a national mega-project. They also result from the accompanying media attention that temporarily places the host in the global spotlight. MSE hosting opportunities are invariably presented as a means of attaining a range of social, political and economic benefits, particularly for the host communities, who customarily are the most directly impacted by delivery of such projects (Dowse 2014; Lindsay 2014). While the socio-economic and political utility of these events has been appreciated for some time, the associated delivery processes also have an established history of raising social justice concerns (Adams and Piekarz 2015; Amnesty International 2013; Brackenridge et al. 2013; Butler and Aicher 2015; COHRE 2007; Finkel 2015).[1]

The lack of effective processes to deal with concerns generated by MSE hosting processes is also evident in contemporary calls by social justice groups, like the Sports and Rights Alliance, for MSE owners to establish a human and social rights framework to protect and promote the interests of those impacted by event delivery processes.[2] Some positive progress has occurred, for example, the International Olympic Committee (IOC) has recently incorporated human rights principles in its Host City Contract, while The Fédération Internationale de Football Association (FIFA) has recognized the United Nations Guiding Principles on Business and Human Rights.[3] However, meaningful outcomes are yet to be identified and the sincerity of event owners to see past their own, predominantly financial, interests remains in doubt.

In part, this slow response could be attributed to the weaknesses in the current knowledge base informing public policy about the actual outcomes of these events, and what an adequate and effective response might entail. This gap is likely to be linked to the historical dominance of the economic justification for hosting which was frequently based on pre-event predictions, rarely followed up by post event evaluations (Coalter 2012). Consequently, there is a great deal of information available on the economic potential of MSEs; much of which actually contests the positive claims made (Feddersen, Grotzinger, and Maennig 2009; de Nooij, van den Berg, and Koopmans 2010). This is not to suggest that there is no support for the possibility of economic benefit (Gratton, Dobson, and Shibli 2001), but the overall message is that realizing it is extremely challenging and will be especially difficult for some hosts. These challenges arise from the contextual sensitivity of event impacts and outcomes, which means that the socio-political and economic environment of the host is an important consideration when seeking to determine what these might be.

It is therefore, unsurprising that concerns have been raised over the relatively recent relocation of events to developing countries which, by their nature, frequently lack the economic, political and social stability of the traditional industrialized host (Matheson and Baade 2004). This contextual difference is important as the absence of this stability, along with invariably lower levels of the organizational and physical infrastructure required for delivery, complicates the achievement of positive outcomes because it makes hosting far more expensive and resource intensive. The expected return on investment for these hosts is also questioned, particularly with respect to the associated infrastructure development and its longer term social value. The recent media images of derelict Olympic stadia in Brazil are a case in point (The Guardian 2017).

The prevalence of negative social outcomes for MSE projects has inevitably drawn attention to the ethical responsibilities of event owners who award their events on the basis of a competitive bidding process. This paper is concerned with exploring debates around whether it is ethically responsible for developing countries to be awarded hosting rights for MSEs when event owners know that, in these countries, community rights and interests are unlikely to have a well-functioning protective framework, public resources are insufficient for existing social priorities and, consequently, vulnerable communities are likely to be placed unnecessarily at risk. Conversely, why these areas seek to host in the first place, especially given the more limited potential for positive social and economic outcomes to be achieved, also needs extrapolating. Both of these questions need to be addressed in order to return to the ethical dilemma of whether, for example, developing countries ought to be protected *from themselves* by event owners through the act of withholding hosting rights. Because, perhaps, if the aims of these hosts can be understood and the reasons why they may or may not be delivered on are recognized, it will be possible to consider whether an ethically driven prohibition on hosting in developing country contexts is fair and justifiable or, whether an appropriate answer for ethical considerations might lie elsewhere.

Sport events, Westernization and the 'non-West'

Events are embedded within the socio-cultural milieus of their host communities. Many of the world's international sporting events, staged since the Second World War, have predominantly emerged and been hosted within Western Europe, North America and Australia. This is, in part, due to the success and growth within these post war nations' economies. These regions of the world, collectively known as the 'developed' or 'Western' world, have developed a series of value systems over what sport is, how and where it should be played and, more importantly to this paper, how and where their associated events ought to be hosted.

International sports governing bodies for the majority of 'major' sports, such as association football, cricket, rugby and tennis, were founded in Western nations and so were also loosely based around Western values. This provided the basis for the structural dominance evident today, as Gupta (2009, 1779) argues 'Because Western nations were the founder members of most international sporting associations they dominated these bodies and set the rules for a sport, dominated its finances, and determined the location of major international events'. This dominance notwithstanding, there is a clear trend towards many 'emerging' regions outside of the Western world hosting, and/or actively seeking to host, international sporting events (Russell et al. 2014). A result of which, as Little (1995) wrote, mega-events,

> Have brought the issues of world justice to the fore of an international political arena long dominated by the self-serving discourse of the world's major industrial powers. (Little 1995, 265)

MSEs have been staged in non-Western countries for some time. For example: Tokyo Olympics, 1964; Mexico Olympics, 1968; Seoul Olympics, 1988; FIFA men's World Cup in Uruguay 1930, Brazil, 1950, Mexico 1986, Japan/South Korea, 2002, South Africa, 2010 and Brazil, 2014. However, for many, the 2008 Beijing Olympic and Paralympic Games set in motion a new social and political agenda for considering the role of non-Western nations on the major international sports events circuit (Palmer 2013). Russell and O'Connor (2013) suggest that the 'success' of Beijing has encouraged other non-Western nations/cities to announce to the IOC their credentials, willingness and readiness to 'bid' to be host cities for future Olympics. However, the current trend may reflect the development of events as a benchmark of development status because to host is considered 'normal practice' for States at a certain level of development. Certainly, it appears possible that the current volume of events held annually means that they no longer easily perform the historical role as marker of distinction in the global marketplace of cities as perhaps they once did.

Indeed, emerging nations from Asia, South America and the Middle East are now actively seeking, and are being courted by event owners and organizers, to be potential future hosts and venues for all types of international sporting events; many of which attract global media audiences (Russell et al. 2014). Countries such as China (Beijing Olympics and Paralympics, 2008; India (Commonwealth Games 2010), Bahrain (Formula One – annual), Russia (men's UEFA Champions League Final, 2010, 2014 Winter Olympics) and Brazil (men's FIFA World Cup, 2014 and Olympic and Paralympic Games, 2016) have all recently staged major sporting events.

This global shift in the hosting of international sporting events outside of the West is set to continue. For example, the men's FIFA Football World Cup will be hosted by Russia in 2018 and Qatar in 2022 respectively. Bang (2011, 1) suggests that 'the biggest events are leaving Europe and North America'. Evidence of this shift can be provided by the Danish Institute for Sports Studies Research which predicts that only 23% of major international events, such as the Olympic and Paralympic Games and world championship tournaments in football, athletics and swimming, will be held within Western countries after 2010. The remaining 77% of these events will be held within countries from the Middle East, Asia, Africa (south of the Sahara Desert) and Central/South America (Bang 2011).

This shifting pattern can be conceptualized through the idea of 'post-Westernization' (Rumford 2007). For Rumford this shift is not simply about the decreasing salience of the idea of the West as a reference point for political identification and global leadership, rather, it can be characterized through a series of processes. Firstly, he suggests that post-Westernization signals the increasing 'lack of unity within those countries formerly considered to have a common "Western" world view' (205). Secondly, post-Westernization signifies the co-existence of multiple 'modernities' – Western, post-communist, Islamic – as opposed to an assumed dominance of the West over the rest. Finally, post-Westernization involves recognition of a 'new East' capable of 'shaping global affairs previously seen as the preserve of the West' (206).

Viewed through the lens of the relocation of MSE, the reality of post-Westernization appears further away than it may actually seem because this development presents international sports organizations and their commercial sponsors with opportunities to make significant economic gains by, for example, accessing new markets, while the associated costs are borne by a host ill-equipped to bear them. The greatest irony to this relationship is that awarding the event to those developing contexts can be perceived as justice for the historically marginalized when it could equally be presented as an opaque tool of exploitation, which offers up scarce resources, and may additionally complicate social and economic development in these areas.

Ultimately, debate continues as to what benefit(s) the staging or hosting of a MSE can actually bring to a country or a city, especially one in the developing world. While it is frequently suggested that hosting opportunities will facilitate much needed social development within the host city/country, the counter position is that their utility is rather to project symbolically a message of parity to the international community. For example, Darnell (2012, 105) argues that, 'sports mega-events ... are used to showcase successful development, particularly for States struggling for legitimacy within competitive globalisation'.

Whilst mega-events clearly present opportunities for development, crucially, the ways in which rights to host are contested, how they are allocated and subsequently, how they are expected to be delivered, are judged according to Western standards. For Hayes and Karamichas (2012, 6), such Western-centrism raises the question of homogenization and cultural standardization, or 'rather the projection of a Western, liberal model of social relations on local host communities'. This begs the question of whether we are in fact witnessing a shifting locus of power after all. That MSEs are being hosted in developing countries with greater frequency is indisputable, however it remains the case that MSE are surrounded by Western logics over their production and delivery which, in many ways, reaffirms, rather than challenges, Western hegemony.

Ethical concerns for the impacts of hosting

The general destabilization of the economic case for hosting MSEs has prompted greater attention on the non-economic opportunities presented by event initiatives, regardless of who the aspirant host is (Chalip 2006; Maennig and Porche 2008). Within or alongside this there has also been a noticeable rise in the attention given to the social cost of delivering an event which hitherto received relatively little attention. For example, research commissioned to inform a joint Dutch – Belgium bid for the 2018 and 2022 men's FIFA Football World Cups drew attention to the absence of a comprehensive and evidence-based approach to evaluating the implications of hosting, particularly with respect to social costs (de Nooij, van den Berg, and Koopmans 2010). This gap suggests that there are a number of governments that have pursued such 'opportunities' without the knowledge required to understand how the event will impact their communities.

Developments in media technology mean that it is now difficult to ignore or conceal the social impacts of hosting projects. In recent years there have been numerous reports and media footage of harm linked to event delivery processes and associated protest (Broudehoux 2012; Lamond and Spracklen 2014). There are continuing debates about the relationship between human rights, social justice issues and events, for example, controversies surrounding the rights of migrant workers in Qatar (2022) and questions of gay rights in Russia (2014) to name a few (see Dowse, Powell, and Weed 2017). It is also possible that the enhanced profile of these issues is a feature of the relocation of mega-events to developing countries. Here, the capacity to absorb the effects of event delivery emerge into sharper focus because, for example, the infrastructure development often perceived as causing the diversion of scarce public funding away from social priorities is likely to have more limited social value and the effects of such diversion more obvious. In such circumstances the MSE becomes the focus for displays of public protest as was witnessed in Brazil in the preparation periods leading to the 2014 men's FIFA Football World Cup and the 2016 Olympic and Paralympic Games (Butler and Aicher 2015).

Growing alongside (and possibly as a consequence of) the increased profile of the negative impacts of event hosting is a growing demand for public influence in the decision to pursue an award. This is evident in the use of referendums to determine whether bid ambitions carry popular support and the results of referendums held in Krakow (2014), Boston (2015) and Hamburg (2015) confirm that this is not guaranteed. However, while civic engagement in the decision-making process is encouraging, it is not clear that the ability to influence relevant decision-making processes extends into the event preparation period if the event is awarded. What is clear is that momentum is growing for both event owners and governments to be made accountable for the impacts of hosting and also for the degree to which outcomes match the promises made (Cornelissen 2012; Dowse 2014).

Given the high profile problems associated with MSEs, is it fair to suggest that aspirant hosts are aware that these initiatives carry a range of risks. What is less clear is how far those in the related political and policy-making circles are aware of the true nature of the event potential in terms of the goals that are realizable and how they might be realized. It is important therefore, that any decision towards hosting is well informed. Research into the 2010 men's FIFA Football World Cup suggests that knowledge concerning very fundamental issues, such as how delivering the event in line with the event owner's wishes and the terms and conditions agreed through the contractual process would constrain activity to achieve local policy goals, varied tremendously across many relevant decision-making networks (Dowse 2014). It was equally true that very specific political and international relations goals existed and it appeared likely that even if at national level there was complete knowledge of these constraints, these drivers would have outweighed such considerations. While as a case study it would be inappropriate to generalize the findings of the South African experience to all developing contexts, key aspects of these findings are offered for consideration.

Understanding the political support for the 2010 men's FIFA Football World Cup hosting project

One of the key features of South Africa's policy ambitions for the 2010 men's FIFA Football World Cup was the foreign policy goal of improving the country's status and position with the international and regional political elite. An important dimension of this expectation was that hosting would improve the ability to pursue and defend national objectives and interests in the future. In part, this expectation was grounded in the belief that the event would convey the symbolic message that the country and, by association, continent, had achieved globally recognized standards of development and deserved to be taken seriously in/by the international community.

This expectation has to be understood in relation to the positioning of developing countries within the international community as subordinate to developed industrialized nations. It also has to be understood in relation to South Africa's unfortunate historical legacy of apartheid which has weakened the country's regional standing and which continues to constrain its ability to pursue regional leadership ambitions (Adebajo, Adedeji, and Landsberg 2007). This ambition was clearly set out by former President, Thabo Mbeki, in a State of the Nation address:

> In the next few months South Africa will launch its bid to host the 2010 Soccer World Cup. Government wishes to assure our Soccer World Cup Bid Committee of our fullest support. … We are certain of victory this time around, a victory that will be for all Africa … as African's to host the Cricket World Cup, like the President's Golf Cup later this year, communicates the

message that we are not wrong when we said that this, the 21st century, will be an African Century. (South Africa: The Presidency 2003a)

The ambition was also re-stated by then Deputy President, Jacob Zuma, at the handover of the bid book:

Africa clearly continues to move away from the fringes, and is asserting her rightful place among other regions of the world … in 2010, Africa will take the stage and rightly so give the positive developments already in place in the continent … It is very important that all should realize that the time has come for Africa to play its part. (South Africa: The Presidency 2003b)

The underlying message in these statements was that South Africa and Africa, as political entities, are set on the outskirts of the international community and do not enjoy a parity of recognition as a consequence. They also confirm that the South African government perceived the hosting initiative as an opportunity to enhance both status and role as a means of developing from its peripheral status on a global stage. This suggests that in order to evaluate the ethical considerations of hosting projects, attention should be paid to exploring the basis and legitimacy of such beliefs and, moreover, whether hosting projects may be an effective means of addressing the challenges observed. To understand this further, we must acknowledge the role of the State in event hosting.

In terms of International Relations theory the State is recognized as the principal actor within the international community and, conceptually, is expected to be an effective service and security provider for its citizens. For this reason, these attributes are linked to internal and external perceptions of capacity, legitimacy and citizen's identification (Van de Walle and Scott 2011). By virtue of constitutional independence, the State is, theoretically, a sovereign entity without internal equal or external superior. The government alone holds the authority to define and implement domestic laws and policies and those which govern foreign engagement and the limitations on the extent of its own authority. In practice, the international community reflects a significant diversity in terms of this sovereign capacity which is reflected in a power configuration between States invariably described as being between the developed North and developing South, the First and Third World or West and non-West (Gupta 2009). Understanding where a State is located in this classification is important because to be defined as Southern, developing, Third World or non-Western, like those States in Latin America or Africa, reflects a position of subordination in relation to Northern, developed, First World or Western States like the United States of America and the United Kingdom. The basis of this positioning is not theoretical. The North/South, First/Third, developed/developing, West/non-West divide is grounded in a history of colonial or imperial domination and, more recently, the emergence of new States through, for example, the territorial break up of Eastern Europe. This history has enabled 'developed' States to consolidate extensive control over key resource channels in the global economy which, in turn maintains their hegemonic position.

We acknowledge that our use of the terms 'West', 'non-West', 'developed', 'developing' etc., are highly problematic and are not easily applied in all contexts. For example, in the case of MSEs, the likes of Bahrain, United Arab Emirates (UAE), Oman, Qatar and Iran are proving to be attractive hosts for staging a range of international sporting events. Financially, these States are wealthier than many within Western Europe and therefore, the financial case can easily be made for staging MSEs here. But what for their socio-cultural 'development'? Their questionable human rights records complicate the issue further and, in so doing, create the additional complexity for scholars, event owners, organizers and other stakeholders of those States which we might describe as 'in-between'.

In essence, newer States have joined an established system with a recognized right to equality, but on the basis of disadvantageous power relations, which undermines this equality in practice. It is therefore, no surprise that improving the capacity to access and influence the 'core' is a frequent foreign policy concern because until this happens, and greater parity is recognized, they will remain marginalized on the periphery or semi-periphery of international relations (Schwengel 2008). These policy goals are incredibly salient when thinking about the engagement of developing or emerging powers with MSEs because these events are hugely symbolic undertakings which are perceived to convey messages of national identity, legitimacy and capability to a domestic and foreign audience. Sports events in particular, provide citizens with opportunities to come together in a visible, collective expression of a national identity and because this is relatively rare in modern societies they offer States the opportunity to project powerful symbols of nationhood (Dashper, Fletcher, and McCullough 2014). The perceived value of this symbolic messaging may outweigh their financial implications and, for this reason, the *irrationality* of investment in an event with limited potential for a substantive economic return can be considered rather rational, especially in countries with weak or limited international profile and influence, with deeply divided societies, or with histories of internal division and conflict.

The variable outcomes of MSEs with respect to economic and social development, image and reputation highlights that hosting initiatives are a possible poisoned chalice. Whether a State (developing or otherwise) should host a MSE is a legitimate question and the answer to this question ought to be made on the basis of an informed understanding of the ways in which their individual context will be impacted by the delivery processes associated with the event, as well as, the goals sought. For this responsible approach to move forward there has to be more clarity/honesty from the hosts about the goals themselves, especially because *promoted*, *perceived* and *actual* goals are not necessarily the same thing. This is clear in research into the economic dimensions of hosting initiatives, which shows that, not only is it hard to achieve an economic return on investment, but also that the key policy-makers are likely to be aware that this is the case (Horne 2004; de Nooij, van den Berg, and Koopmans 2010). This suggests that economic concerns have not been the main motivation for these hosts and that policy statements are used primarily to gain the necessary public support to pursue hosting opportunities. For these more socio-cultural dimensions, the core question of whether MSEs can and do offer States a return on investment, which balances the associated risk and costs, remains as salient as it is for the economic dimension. However, evaluating the wisdom of policy decisions grounded in these objectives is infinitely harder than evaluating economic dimensions. This may be the reason why there are fewer studies in this area and consequently, less empirical evidence of the outcomes gained.

What is known about the potential for image and reputation-based dividends is that, like economic, the opportunities are primarily grounded in the ability to capture global attention and elevate popular interest in the host nation. This potential is identified in the pre-event and post-event phases as well as games time. Through this, MSEs are expected to help States develop, or consolidate, a 'brand' (Sturm 2015). The perceived 'brand' of a country is important, for as previously discussed, the power and status of a State is influenced by how it is perceived and understood by others, and this will be informed by the views and stereotypes held about it. Mega-events can support positive image and reputation development because they offer opportunities to project positive imagery. Moreover, in those instances where a State is attempting to overturn negative perceptions, event hosting can help demonstrate distance travelled from 'then' through to 'now'. The South Korean government displayed this political ambition through the 2002 men's FIFA Football World Cup which was expected to help the country 'rebrand itself as a leading economy after the Asian economic crisis of the late 1990s' (Horne 2004, 1244).

While the successful delivery of a MSE that meets and reflects global standards of development certainly ought to enhance the reputation and image of the host, the positive potential in this area may be less than anticipated. This disjoint reflects the difficulties inherent in changing established perceptions and underpins the need for strategic and long-term investment in image and reputation development. Consequently, MSEs are only likely to be effective as a tool of image and reputation change if they are used as part of a broader nation-branding strategy. Indeed, evidence suggests that image and reputation change is unlikely to occur if the event is the focus of a temporary marketing campaign (Anholt 2011). In addition, event-led makeovers are also problematic as they risk exposing the host to unhelpful media projections that reinforce negative stereotypes or may focus attention on political activity and social situations that may compromise positive reputations (Dimeo and Kay 2004; Finlay and Xin 2010; Palmer 2013). Problems in the event delivery process are also likely to receive extensive coverage which may inhibit the positive images hosts seek to convey. For example, media reports of the 2010 Commonwealth Games in New Delhi which documented unsanitary living conditions and infrastructure failures, like the collapse of a pedestrian bridge, were invariably unaligned to the image the hosts sought to project (Curi, Knijnik, and Mascarenhas 2011).

Anticipated positive outcomes, with respect to image and reputational change may be difficult to achieve because media coverage tends to rely on imagery and narratives that are informed by and reinforce existing stereotypes (Darcy 2003; Dimeo and Kay 2004). This implies that the positive marketing potential of events is likely to be lower for countries that are associated with negative stereotypes and, in turn, are also in greatest need of re-imaging support. In the main, these countries are likely to be the more newly established and which do not currently possess the levels of political, social and economic stability of their peers, thus identifying them as different and potentially less valuable. As a result, Dimeo and Kay (2004) suggest that developing countries and former colonies have less capacity to control media discourses, and are additionally challenged by the need to counter the use of colonial terms of reference and stereotypes in media reports. Darnell (2014, 1000) supports this position and suggests that popular representations of sport and events 'can serve to secure the innocence and benevolence of global sport for Western audiences while insulating them from, and therefore solidifying, the political economy of unequal development.'

However, any attempts to make sweeping generalizations about the hosting capacity of developing nations are not advised because developed nations are by no means insulated from negative and potentially damaging media coverage. For example, a comparative analysis of the coverage of the 2006 and 2010 men's FIFA Football World Cups held in Germany and South Africa, respectively, found that the tone of reporting was remarkably similar, despite the fact that Germany is a developed country and not a former colony, while South Africa is a developing economy with a history of colonial control (Media Tenor 2010). Interviews carried out with reporters as part of the study into the South African experience explored this feature of the findings and feedback received suggested a level of benevolence in reporting of the 2010 event which may have reflected a general consensus to recognize the additional challenges faced by South Africa.[4] It was additionally suggested that this benevolent approach was not witnessed in the case of Germany and would be unlikely for future developed country hosts. However, interpreting this as wholly positive for South Africa as it appears prima facie would be ill-advised. Indeed, such an approach from the media arguably does little to challenge Orientalist discourses surrounding the backwardness and organizational inefficiencies of developing nations and, as such, could have the opposite effect of reinforcing neo-colonial rhetoric of Western paternal dominance and superiority. Ultimately, this means that while event-hosting may support positive image development, as part of a wider programme of image improvement there are significant risks involved; risks that political stakeholders may neither fully appreciate nor have the capacity to manage.

Within the domestic polity, events are perceived as capable of supporting the consolidation of political legitimacy because locating an event in a country signals that the host has been recognized as the legitimate territorially bound political authority (Levermore 2004).[5] This is important because external recognition confers legitimacy on claims to statehood and this recognition may have internal significance because they provide positive collective 'moments' that can foster sentiments of unity across divided domestic populations. The 1995 men's Rugby World Cup in South Africa illustrates these possibilities and is well known for a perceived nation-building effect. However, despite receiving plaudits for this nation-building impact, how meaningful the effect was is debated and the associated discussions question whether the collective euphoria identified should be interpreted as social cohesion or as a temporary display of positive emotions inflated by the media and emotional heat of the event (Grundlingh 1998; Hendricks 2008).

Core to the concerns about the nation-building potential of sport events is that the organizers are primarily concerned with event delivery and not necessarily the social problems that exist internally. Moreover, rather than alleviating these problems, sports events may risk exacerbating social divides by emphasising existing inequalities and diverting resources from other social priorities (Butler and Aicher 2015; Hylton and Morpeth 2012). The pressures created by hosting an event with a fixed deadline for delivery, can result in the suppression of civil rights and undermine the perceived legitimacy of the host government. There are examples of suppression in established democratic States, including Australia and the UK (Lindsay 2014; Nauright 2004), which makes the trend for events to be hosted more regularly in non-established democracies and emerging States like Russia, Qatar and South Africa (where civil rights are inconsistently enjoyed or protected) particularly worrying.

MSEs are globally popular commercial spectacles that offer numerous opportunities to advance political ambitions. Although marketed on the basis of their economic potential, weaknesses in the economic evidence base suggests that broader socio-political dimensions are more influential motivators of political support. Problematically, information regarding the actual impact of MSEs in terms of nation-building, and the social outcomes that lie below, is sparse. In part, this is because there are few agreed proxies for measuring such impacts and those that are recognized tend to be temporary. Moreover, these non-economic drivers are obfuscated by the need to justify the public expenditure involved, particularly as positive 'intangible' outcomes are difficult to demonstrate and quantify. This does not mean that they are unrealisable. MSEs have a potentially unique capacity to capture global attention and elevate popular interest in a country over a sustained period of time. In the context of national interests, defined in terms of enhanced foreign and domestic policy capacity, the political opportunities that hosting presents are extensive and broad-ranging. For these reasons, events are attractive policy options for all countries, but potentially more so for the political elite in contexts where domestic structures and capacities require development and where international influence or commercial engagement is weak. These are certainly characteristics of the developing country hosts that are now competing successfully to secure hosting rights.

This raises the possibility that, rather than the opportunity to gain specific benefits linked to the event, the contemporary demand for hosting rights in developing country contexts is a consequence of political developments in international relations. These developments include a shift in political and economic power away from the global North or 'West' and demands for greater equality of opportunity and parity of status by emerging economies. Explored through this perspective, it is possible that hosting ambitions are located within a broad and over-arching political ambition to re-define relations in the international community and, in so doing, gain access to the political and economic opportunities held by those occupying the 'core' (those traditionally described as the 'West') of international relations.

Event owners are amenable to this development because a shift in location offers a valuable opportunity to access new and developing consumer markets on a proportionately low risk basis (Russell et al. 2014). Indeed the potential return from an emerging country host could be extensive, particularly if organizational inexperience in the management of mega-projects and weaknesses in governmental structures increase vulnerability to exploitation through, for example, disadvantageous contracting processes (Dowse 2014). However, it could also be argued that the relocation of events to developing countries offers opportunities to maintain existing power structures of dominance by the core over the periphery by providing access to political and economic resources under the guise of 'justice' for development.

What then are the ethical questions?

The formal sovereignty of States within the international community renders a universal exclusion of certain polities from the global competition inappropriate. Such prohibition would be discriminatory, while at the same time deny these countries the opportunity to explore alternative means of addressing domestic and foreign policy concerns – and particularly those that reflect the structural disadvantages of the international community. It would also reinforce the positioning of countries as subordinate and subject to a form of neo-colonial control.

However, this is not to suggest that the processes currently in place for awarding events could not be improved or that the policy decisions made by political leaders with respect to MSEs are necessarily well-informed. It is reasonably safe to assume that international sport governing bodies like FIFA and the IOC welcome the move of events to developing country contexts, not only for altruistic ideals of sharing opportunities, but also for the commercial opportunities presented in terms of accessing new markets. Research by Dowse into the South African experience also suggests that this relationship can be tainted by the perception that the governing body is exploiting their host's weaknesses in ways that reflect the disadvantages experienced as a result of their subordinate position within the international community generally. This exploitative side of the relationship may not be immediately apparent. For example, initially, FIFA's introduction in 2000 of the policy of rotation and the award of the event to South Africa was positioned by the government as justice gained for a continent historically marginalized by the international community.[6] However, as the process of delivery unfolded it appeared that, rather than justice, the event became a mechanism for paternal exploitation by FIFA. Much of this was linked to the contractual obligations associated with the event which were poorly understood initially, and which had debilitating implications. It also appeared that political sensitivities to perceptions of incompetence and the desire for international approval weakened South Africa's negotiating position in relation to FIFA, with the net effect being a compression of the ability to achieve foreign and domestic policy priorities, whether directly associated with the event or not. The case of South Africa is but one example that clearly illustrates the complexities involved in hosting MSEs; complexities that, evidence suggests, are exacerbated when considered in developing contexts.

How we manage the demands and expectations of governing bodies and event own-ers with the host project is an important area within event studies that has not generally received a great deal of attention. If we centralize ethics as an event host consideration, this is a significant omission. Indeed, that we know very little about the relationships between hosts and key stakeholders raises a number of ethical issues regarding how governments may lose control of the parameters of event delivery in ways that compromise the outcomes sought through the hosting initiative. It may also be the case, as we have suggested for the men's FIFA Football World Cup in South Africa, that international sports organizations may gain power, albeit temporarily, within a sovereign nation State through the hosting process in ways that could be considered comparable to that held by another sovereign State with greater power resources. More generally, these considerations bring to light the possibility that States new to hosting global mega-events have very limited understanding of what they are getting involved in and, as a result, might be seduced by what become unrealisable opportunities, much to the detriment of local communities' everyday lives. Such a situation may derive from a governing body's control of the management processes associated with the event and an historical lack of inter-State knowledge exchange. The ability to assert such dominance with little resistance from the host might be reflective of a lack of State-confidence to negotiate with a body that effectively holds the keys to Pandora's Box and the opportunities therein.

Conclusion

Given the significant financial investment required to successfully host a MSE, it is absolutely essential that all parties involved in the process sufficiently understand and appreciate the opportunities and pitfalls associated. We know that, by their very nature, developing nations are less affluent and arguably less prepared to deliver large scale sports events than developed nations. Within developing contexts the cost of hosting and risk of failing to achieve sought outcomes is likely to be far higher than for events held in the developed world. Therefore, it is appropriate to ask, 'are governing bodies, when equipped with this knowledge, ethically obliged to withhold hosting rights from developing countries?'

Some might argue that this is the responsible thing to do. Palmer (2013) reasserts that a major challenge facing organizers in developing contexts is ensuring that they do not fall victim to Global North/First World/developed/Western perceptions that they are boxing above their weight. In other words, they must ensure they succeed – otherwise they will reinforce the perception that they are not developed enough to host an event of such magnitude. The failure of one event has an influential demonstration effect for other developing nations. Palmer suggests there is an element of 'I told you so' amongst developed nations when developing nations either struggle or fail. She warns that the obvious solution for avoiding such a situation is for developing nations to invest disproportionately in the event. For example, the original budget for the 2010 Commonwealth Games in New Delhi was US$1.3 billion. This was reported to have mushroomed to US$15 billion, which was seven times more expensive than Melbourne in 2006, leading Majumdar and Mehta to describe the event as 'by far and away the most expensive games in history' (cited in Palmer 2013, 116). Palmer goes on to argue that this is because there is a tendency amongst developing nations to, not only aim to *equal* the achievements of their developed counterparts, they wish to *outdo* them. Given that success is invariably judged in relation to previous hosts' performances it is likely that all hosts seek to outdo their predecessor, whether they are developed or not, but the implications of exceeding the delivery capabilities of a developed country has far deeper resource implications; especially for countries which are starting from a lower level.

This notwithstanding, denying sovereign States the right to make their own decisions would appear to compound the low status of countries that MSE hosting is perceived to address. For this reason, it seems sensible to suggest that a more appropriate response to the ethical dilemma of hosting rights is not to withhold them from States at lower levels of development, but rather to support them meet their goals and protect national interests. This would involve: (1) improving understanding of the policy outcomes sought and why; (2) raising awareness of the problems that could arise in achieving these outcomes; (3) more effectively managing the demands that event owners and governing bodies place on hosts. The bigger question here is *who should be responsible for this*?

Developing countries are on the periphery of the international community and are frequently subjugated. Mega-event hosting offers an opportunity to gain recognition from and access to the developed world, if only symbolically. Given that events have historically been hosted by developed countries, much of what is known reflects delivery in developed country contexts which, by association, reflects the world view of the specific developed country and its global position. Given the substantial difference, a simple transfer of lessons learned and resultant expectations from the developed country experience is inappropriate in ways that parallel debates concerning 'universal' and 'relative' approaches to human rights and the standards and policies designed to achieve them (Bentley 2005).

Further, there is also the issue that despite laudable claims, the primary interest of the event owners is the delivery of an event. It remains the case that hosts – particularly those in the developing world – are potentially vulnerable to exploitation by the event owner. Ultimately though, any associated social and political impacts to the hosts remain the host's responsibility. The point is not to suggest that this obviates the duty to protect citizens or that the capacity and priority for doing so should not be a fundamental piece of the award criteria. However, this is a qualitatively different consideration to the question of whether the capacity to make that decision should be denied to them based on an external evaluation of their capacity to meet externally determined judgements on social impact thresholds which appears, prima facie, to be denying an opportunity for sovereign decision-making.

It seems reasonable to suggest that, due to the imperatives of global sport and the need to attract new audiences and investors, there is a need to expand sporting events into hitherto uncharted territories. This will require a reconsideration of many of the hegemonic ideological assumptions around which international sports events are currently conceptualized (Russell et al. 2014). Palmer (2013) argues that a central feature of global sports events policy is the Westernization of cultural mores and values in non-Western host cities. The 2010 men's FIFA Football World Cup acts as a case in point. Dowse (2014) argues that throughout South Africa's journey to host the event, the imperative to satisfy FIFA's various contractual demands regarding financing and infrastructure, amongst many others, created a situation in which national and local interests were highly vulnerable to those of the event. For example, the priorities of the event owner, in terms of stadia location in Cape Town, where the decision to build a stadium at Green Point rather than Athlone, ran in counter to local development priorities. The subordination of national interests to accommodate mega-event prerogatives is significant because the rhetoric surrounding MSEs is that they will act as a catalyst for much needed social improvements.

We acknowledge that the content of this paper is preliminary. Our intention was not necessarily to provide answers to our observations. Rather, our intention was to provoke others to engage in work on this topic. At the very least, our aim was to shed light on some of the back stage, anticipatory concerns that surround hosting MSEs in developing or non-Western contexts. In so doing, we hope these are now front stage and will be interrogated further.

Notes

1. Despite the established nature of these concerns, reports from the most recently held events in Brazil, the 2014 men's FIFA Football World Cup and the 2016 Summer Olympic Games, suggest that an effective response to these concerns has yet to be established (cf. Marinho, Campagnani, and Cosentino 2014, 37–40).
2. The Sport and Rights Alliance is a coalition of leading NGOs, sports organizations and trade unions. It was founded in early 2015 to address the decision-makers of international sports mega-events to introduce measures to ensure these events are always organized in a way that respects human rights (including labour rights), the environment and anti-corruption requirements at all stages of the process (for more information, visit: http://www.sportandhumanrights.org/wordpress/index.php/2015/07/06/sport-and-rights-alliance/.
3. See http://www.fifa.com/about-fifa/news/y=2015/m=7/news=fifa-executive-committee-sets-presidential-election-for-26-february-20-2666448.html for more information.
4. Interviews with UK and international based sport reporters conducted by Dowse in 2010.
5. Outside of political organizations like the United Nations, the membership of international sports organisations is one of the few ways in which the status of statehood may be recognized.
6. In 2000 the FIFA Executive Committee voted for the men's World Cup tournament to be rotated from continent to continent. As from 2018, the hosting of the event will cease to be rotated.

Disclosure statement

No potential conflict of interest was reported by the author.

References

Adams, A., and M. Piekarz. 2015. "Sport Tourism and Human Rights: Positive or Negative Erosion?" *Journal of Policy Research in Tourism, Leisure and Events* 10: 1–17 doi:10.1080/19407963.2014.997864.

Adebajo, A., A. Adedeji, and C. Landsberg. 2007. "Introduction." In *South Africa in Africa: The Post-apartheid Era*, edited by A. Adebajo, A. Adedeji and C. Landsberg, 17–39. Scottsville: University of KwaZulu-Natal Press.

Amnesty International. 2013. *The Dark Side of Migration: Spotlight on Qatar's Construction Sector Ahead of the World Cup*. London: Amnesty International.

Anholt, S. 2011. "Beyond the Nation Brand: The Role of Image and Identity in International Relations." *Exchange* 2: 6–12.

Bang, S. 2011. *Western Countries are Losing the Race for Major Sporting Events* [Online] Accessed May 7, 2013. http://www.playthegame.org/news/detailed/western-countries-are-losing-the-race-for-major-sporting-events-5156.html

Bentley, K. A. 2005. "Can There be any Universal Children's Rights?" *International Journal of Human Rights* 9 (1): 107–123. doi: 10.1080/13642980500032370.

Brackenridge, C., S. Palmer-Felgate, D. Rhind, L. Hills, T. Kay, L. Tiivas, L. Faulkner, and I. Lindsay. 2013. *Child Exploitation and the FIFA World Cup: A Review of Risks and Protective Interventions*. Brunel: Brunel Centre for Sport, Health and Wellbeing.

Broudehoux, A. 2012. "Civilizing Beijing: Social Beautification, Civility and Citizenship at the 2008 Olympics." In *Olympic Games, Mega-Events and Civil Societies*, edited by G. Hayes and J. Karamichas, 46–67. Basingstoke: Palgrave Macmillan.

Butler, B., and T. Aicher. 2015. "Demonstrations and Displacement: Social Impact and the 2014 FIFA World Cup." *Journal of Policy Research in Tourism, Leisure and Events* 7 (3): 299–313. doi: 10.1080/19407963.2014.997436.

Chalip, L. 2006. "Towards Social Leverage of Sports Events." *Journal of Sport & Tourism* 11 (2): 109–127. doi: 10.1080/14775080601155126.

Coalter, F. 2012. "Sport-in-development: Accountability or Development?" In *Sport and International Development*, edited by R. Levermore and A. Beacom, 55–75. Basingstoke: Palgrave Macmillan.

COHRE. 2007. *Fair Play for Housing Rights: Mega-events – Mega-Events, Olympic Games and Housing Rights*. Geneva: The Centre on Housing Rights and Evictions (COHRE).

Cornelissen, S. 2012. A Delicate Balance: Major Sports Events and Development. In *Sport and international development*, edited by R. Levermore and A. Beacom, 76–97. Basingstoke: Palgrave Macmillan.

Curi, M., J. Knijnik, and G. Mascarenhas. 2011. "The Pan American Games in Rio de Janeiro 2007: Consequences of a sport mega-event in a BRIC country." *International Review for the Sociology of Sport* 46 (2): 140–156. doi: 10.1177/1012690210388461.

Darcy, S. 2003. "The Politics of Disability and Access: The Sydney 2000 Games Experience." *Disability and Society* 18 (6): 737–757. doi: 10.1080/0968759032000119497.

Darnell, S. C. 2012. *Sport for Development and Peace: A Critical Sociology*. London: Bloomsbury.

Darnell, S. C. 2014. "Orientalism through Sport: Towards a Said-ian Analysis of Imperialism and 'Sport for Development and Peace.'" *Sport in Society* 17 (8): 1000–1014. doi: 10.1080/17430437.2013.838349.

Dashper, K., T. Fletcher, and N. McCullough. 2014. Sports Events, Society and Culture. In *Sports Events, Society and Culture*, edited by K. Dashper, T. Fletcher, and N. McCullough, 1–22. London: Routledge.

Dimeo, P., and T. Kay. 2004. "Major Sports Events, Image Projection and the Problems of 'Semi-Periphery': A Case Study of the 1996 South Asia Cricket World Cup." *Third World Quarterly* 25 (7): 1263–1276. doi: 10.1080/014365904200281267.

Dowse, S. 2014. "Knowing the Rules and Understanding the Score: The 2010 FIFA Football World Cup in South Africa." In *Sports Events, Society and Culture*, edited by K. Dashper, T. Fletcher and N. McCullough, 205–220. London: Routledge.

Dowse, S., S. Powell, and M. Weed. 2017. Mega-sporting Events and Children's Rights and Interests – towards a Better Future. *Leisure Studies*. Published online ahead of print, doi: 10.1080/02614367.2017.1347698

Feddersen, A., A. Grotzinger, and W. Maennig. 2009. "Investment in Stadia and Regional Economic Development Evidence from FIFA World Cup 2006" *International Journal of Sport Finance* 4 (4): 221–239.

Finkel, R. 2015. "Introduction: Social Justice and Events-related Policy." *Journal of Policy Research in Tourism, Leisure and Events* 7 (3): 217–219. doi: 10.1080/19407963.2014.995905

Finlay, C., and X. Xin. 2010. "Public Diplomacy Games: a Comparative Study of American and Japanese Responses to the Interplay of Nationalism, Ideology and Chinese Soft Power Strategies around the 2008 Beijing Olympics." *Sport in Society* 13 (5): 876–900. doi: 10.1080/17430431003651115

Fletcher, T., and Dashper, K. 2013 "'Bring on the Dancing Horses!': Ambivalent reporting of Dressage at London 2012". *Sociological Research Online* 18 (2). http://www.socresonline.org.uk/18/2/17.html

Gratton, C., N. Dobson, and S. Shibli. 2001. "The Role of Major Sports Events in the Economic Regeneration of Cities: Lessons from Six World or European Championships." In *Sport in the City: The Role of Sport in Economic and Social Regeneration*, edited by C. Gratton and I. P. Henry, 35–45. London: Routledge.

Grundlingh, A. 1998. "From Redemption to Recidivism? Rugby and Change in South Africa during the 1995 Rugby World Cup and its Aftermath." *Sporting Traditions* 14 (2): 67–86.

Gupta, A. 2009. "The Globalisation of Sports, the Rise of Non-western Nations, and the Impact on International Sporting Events." *The International Journal of the History of Sport* 26 (2): 1779–1790. doi: 10.1080/09523360903172390

Hayes, G., and J. Karamichas, eds. 2012. *Olympic Games, Mega-events and Civil Societies: Globalization, Environment and Resistance*. Basingstoke: Palgrave.

Hendricks, D. J. 2008. The Impact of Mega Sports Events on the Social Fabric of Developing Communities: Dreamfields: Exploiting the Potential of the 2010 FIFA World Cup to Impact Positively on South African Society. Paper presented at The Impact of Mega Sports Events on Development Goals International Symposium, Stellenbosch, March 5–7, 2008. Accessed July 22, 2011. http://www.toolkitsportdevelopment.org/mega-events/html/topic_D10E0070-08F7-48E7-B574-498D57A7B49A_9A33E644-7384-443D-B1C2-D82F67865B35_1.htm

Horne, J. 2004. "The Global Game of Football: The 2002 World Cup and Regional Development in Japan." *Third World Quarterly* 25 (7): 1233–1244. doi: 10.1080/014365904200281249

Hylton, K., and N. D. Morpeth. 2012. "London 2012: 'Race' Matters and the East End." *International Journal of Sport Policy and Politics* 4: 1–18.

Lamond, I. R., and K. Spracklen, eds. 2014. *Protests as Events: Politics, Activism and Leisure*. London: Roman & Littlefield.

Levermore, R. 2004. "Sport's Role in Constructing the "Inter-state" Worldview." In *Sport and international relations: An emerging relationship?*, edited by R. Levermore and A. Budd, 16–30. London: Routledge.

Lindsay, I. 2014. "London 2012: The Rings of Exclusion." In *Sports Events, Society and Culture*, edited by K. Dashper, T. Fletcher and N. L. McCullough, 221–236. London: Routledge.

Little, P. 1995. "Ritual, Power and Ethnography at the Rio Earth Summit." *Critique of Anthropology* 15 (3): 256–283. doi: 10.1177/0308275X9501500303.

Maennig, W., and M. Porche 2008. The Feel-good Effect at Mega Sports Events: Recommendations for Public and Private Administration Informed by the Experience of the FIFA World Cup 2006. *Hamburg Contemporary Economic* Discussions, No. 18[Online] Accessed August 9, 2010. http://www.hced.uni-hamburg.de/WorkingPapers/018.pdf.

Marinho, G., M. Campagnani, and R. Cosentino. 2014. "Brazil." In *World Cup for Whom and for What? A Look upon the Legacy of the World Cups in Brazil, South Africa and Germany*, edited by M. de Paula and D. Bartlet, 12–59. Brasil: Henrich Boll Stiftung.

Matheson, V., and R. Baade. 2004. "Mega-sporting Events in Developing Nations: Playing the Way to Prosperity?" *The South African Journal of Economics* 72 (5): 1085–1095.doi: 10.1111/j.1813-6982.2004.tb00147.x.

Media Tenor. 2010. *WC 2010: Correct Misconceptions? Pre-World Cup Coverage of the Host of WC 2010 (May)*. New York: Media Tenor.

Nauright, J. 2004. "Global Games: Culture, Political Economy and Sport in the Globalised World of the 21st Century." *Third World Quarterly* 25 (7): 1325–1336. doi: 10.1080/014365904200281302

de Nooij, M., M. van den Berg, and C. Koopmans. 2010. Bread or Games? Social Cost-benefit Analysis of the World Cup in the Netherlands. Discussion paper No. 60: SEO Economic Research. Amsterdam [Online] Accessed March 5, 2011. http://www.seo.nl/en/page/article/bread-or-games/

Palmer, C. 2013. *Global Sports Policy*. London: Sage.

Rumford, C. 2007. "More than a Game: Globalization and the Post-westernization of World Cricket." *Global Networks*. 7 (2): 202–214. doi: 10.1111/glob.2007.7.issue-2

Russell, K. A., and N. O'Connor. 2013. "The London 2012 Olympic Games: The Cultural Tourist as a Pillar of Sustainability." In *Cultural Tourism*, edited by R. Raj, K. Griffin and N. Morpeth, 204–211. Wallingford: CABI.

Russell, K., N. O'Connor, K. Dashper, and T. Fletcher. 2014. "Sporting Mega-events and Islam: An Introduction." In *Sports Events, Society and Culture*, edited by K. Dashper., T. Fletcher, and N. McCullough, 189–204. London: Routledge.

Schwengel, H. 2008. "Emerging Powers as Fact and Metaphor: Some European ideas." *Futures* 40: 767–776. doi: 10.1016/j.futures.2008.02.006

Sharpley, R., and P. Stone. 2011. " Socio-cultural Impacts of Events." In *Routledge Handbook of Events*, edited by S. Page and J. Connell, 347–361. London: Routledge.

Sturm, D. 2015. "Fluid Spectator-tourists': Innovative Televisual Technologies, Global Audiences and the 2015 Cricket World Cup." *Comunicazioni Sociali* 2: 230–240.

South Africa: The Presidency (2003a). *State of the Nation Address of the President of South Africa, Thabo Mbeki*, Houses of Parliament, Cape Town, 14 February [Online] Accessed May 5, 2010. http://www.info.gov.za/speeches/2003/03021412521001.htm

South Africa: The Presidency (2003b). J. Zuma: *Handover of SA 2010 Bid Book, 29 September 2003* [Online] Accessed May 5, 2010. http://www.polity.org.za/article/j-zuma-handover-of-sa-2010-bid-book-26092003-2003-09-26

The Guardian. 2017. "Rio's Olympic Venues, Six Months on – in Pictures." [online] Accessed March 21, 2017. https://www.theguardian.com/sport/gallery/2017/feb/10/rios-olympic-venues-six-months-on-in-pictures

Van de Walle, S., and Z. Scott. 2011. "The Political Role of Service Delivery in State-Building: Exploring the Relevance of European History for Developing Countries." *Development Policy Review* 29 (1): 5–21. doi: 10.1111/dpr.2011.29.issue-1

Gulf autocrats and sports corruption: a marriage made in heaven

James M. Dorsey

ABSTRACT

Global soccer and global sports governance have for the past nine years and certainly since a fateful meeting in late 2010 of the executive committee of the Fédération Internationale de Football Association (FIFA), the world soccer body, witnessed crisis after crisis. Invariably the scandals involved various forms of corruption: financial corruption, political corruption or corruption of sporting performance. Gulf autocracies were often at the centre of the financial and political corruption scandals and have in unacknowledged ways served as examples of non-transparent, top-down governance designed to mask first and foremost the inextricable intertwining of politics and sports.

The rise of Gianni Infantino as president of FIFA has led the soccer body to project a new, cleaner era of governance in which the generation of executives loyal to former disgraced president Sepp Blatter were retired and the organization was seen to be tackling financial and performance corruption. In many ways, however, reform of FIFA is comparable to change in the Gulf where autocracies are seeking to upgrade and adjust authoritarian rule to the requirements of the twenty-first century rather than liberalize. Like in the Gulf, reform at FIFA has involved a mix of real and cosmetic change that stopped short of tinkering with political relationships. Yet, it is those relationships that compromise the integrity of sports governance at international, regional and national levels and at times enable other forms of corruption.

The multiple scandals and controversies testify to the little discussed undermining of good governance in sports as a result of an ungoverned relationship between sports and politics and the denial of that relationship by international sports executives and politicians. What many global sports' scandals and controversies have in common is more than a coincidental involvement of Gulf personalities. They reflect the problems involved in a relationship that is allowed to flourish unregulated and unregulated.

A mutually beneficial relationship

Gulf autocrats are well served by the insistence by international sports associations that a Chinese wall divides sports and politics. It allows FIFA to serve as a pillar of autocracy in the soccer-crazy Gulf as well as across the Middle East and North Africa where political control of sports is a tool to garner political support, divert attention away from popular grievances and prevent stadiums from becoming venues of protest. FIFA's selective application of its rules enables the region's autocrats to enhance their international standing, polish their tarnished images, create the leverage that allows them to punch above their weight and manage discontent at home.[1]

Men like Qatari national Mohammed Bin Hammam, the now disgraced former head of the Asian Football Confederation (AFC), a FIFA affiliate, and FIFA executive committee member; Bin Hammam's successor and a member of Bahrain's ruling family, Sheikh Salman Bin Ibrahim Al-Khalifa; and Salman's protector, Kuwaiti Sheikh Ahmad Al-Fahad Al-Ahmed Al-Sabah, a member of the International Olympic Committee (IOC) and FIFA's Council as well as head of the Olympic Council of Asia (OCA), exemplify the intertwining of sports and politics. They are products of autocracies whose rise in international sports was paved in the 1970s when Middle Eastern geopolitics spilt on to the soccer pitch.

At the time, FIFA threatened but failed to follow through on threats to sanction the AFC for its expulsion of Israel as well as Taiwan in violation of the principle of a separation of sports from politics. Ironically, Israel benefitted even though FIFA and the AFC's actions amounted to undeclared support of Middle Eastern autocracy. The policy served to strengthen the region's autocrats whom Israel despite an official state of war long viewed as regimes it could do business with and who were less likely to seek its physical destruction.

FIFA and the AFC's handling of Israel and the Israeli–Palestinian conflict has since come full circle in the wake of the 2011 popular Arab revolts that have rocked the Middle East and mounting international criticism of Israeli policies that among other things hinders the development of Palestinian soccer. After years of failed mediation efforts, FIFA is struggling to fend off attempts to suspend Israel's membership for allowing West Bank settlement teams to play in Israeli leagues.[2]

FIFA's failure to act against the AFC wrote Arab politics into the DNA of Asian soccer and helped shape global soccer's cosiness with autocracy.[3] Politics underwrote the failure. FIFA's failure and the AFC's defiance created the basis for an on-going policy by both organizations that effectively supports autocratic rule by refusing to insist on universal adherence by national associations to the principles, rules and regulations of the global and regional governing bodies.[4]

The failure reverberates in the selective enforcement by FIFA and the AFC of rules and regulations governing the eligibility of clubs to compete in premier leagues and abidance by principles of non-discrimination. Clubs in Iran and Egypt are often government-controlled or owned in violation of single ownership rules and clubs elsewhere in the region have ties or are entities of families ruling with absolute power. Similarly, Iran and Saudi Arabia bar women from entering stadiums where men's competitions are held. Saudi Arabia moreover refuses to ensure that women's sporting rights encompass all disciplines. AFC general secretary Alex Soosay went as far as to defend Iran's ban on women entering stadiums during the Asian Games in Australia in early 2015.[5]

The AFC's intimate association with politics is further highlighted by former secretary general Peter Velappan's glowing description of the group's long-standing efforts to build bridges between feuding parties on the Asian continent such as India and Pakistan, North and South Korea, Iraq and the Gulf states following the 1990 Iraqi invasion of Kuwait, and China and Taiwan.[6]

FIFA and AFC support of autocracy takes on added significance in a world in which the politics of soccer has played an important, if not a key role in the development of various Middle Eastern and North African nations since the late nineteenth and early twentieth centuries. That role is reflected in the fact that a large number of soccer clubs in the region were founded with political associations and continuous efforts by autocratic governments to politically control the game. It is also evident in the politics underlying the Middle East and North Africa's foremost derbies, including Teheran's Esteghlal FC v Persepolis FC, a traditionally leftist opposition club versus one historically associated with Iran's rulers, Amman's Al-Faisali SC v Al-Wehdat SC, a reflection of Jordan's East Bank-Palestinian divide and Cairo's Al Ahli v. Zamalek.[7]

The relationship between Middle Eastern autocracy and global soccer governance is rooted in their similarities and secretive ways that are pockmarked by lack of transparency and accountability. In an electoral message in his first AFC campaign, Salman, a former soccer player, asserted that 'I believe that too many power and political games are affecting the harmony of Asian football when the only game that should matter is the one taking place on football pitches. As leaders in our sport, we must never lose sight of the fact that we are first and foremost servants of the game, at all levels and in all corners of the Asian continent'. Salman listed as his values 'fair play, cooperation, team work, transparency, integrity and passion for the game'.[8]

FIFA's autocratic instincts were put on public display when in 2015, its electoral committee took to task presidential candidate Prince Ali bin Al Hussein of Jordan for criticizing Salman's failure to stand up for detained and abused soccer players in 2011. Nor did it interfere when Salman in 2014 used his position as AFC president to create opportunity to put Bahrain with its severely tarnished image positively on display by moving the confederation's congress from AFC headquarters in Kuala Lumpur to Bahrain. FIFA was also silent when Salman manipulated electoral procedures during the congress to ensure that Ahmad got the FIFA executive committee seat he wanted.[9]

Salman's failure to adhere to his electoral promises and values has contributed to the inability of both the AFC and FIFA to fully put behind them the worst corruption and mismanagement scandal in the history of world soccer even if a number of soccer executives have been sanctioned. In fact, a cleaning of the AFC's house in line with recommendations of an internal audit of the Asian group's finances in 2012 that toppled Bin Hammam, who was in 2013 banned for life from involvement in professional soccer, could have helped spark badly needed reform of the world body.

The audit conducted by PricewaterhouseCooper (PWC) suggested that the AFC under Bin Hammam's management may have been involved in money laundering, tax invasion, bribery, and busting of US sanctions against Iran and North Korea. PwC warned that 'it is our view that there is significant risk that the AFC may have been used as a vehicle to launder funds and that the funds have been credited to the former President (Bin Hammam) for an improper purpose (Money Laundering risk), The AFC may have been used as a vehicle to launder the receipt and payment of bribes'. The audit questioned a $1 billion master rights agreement (MRA) between the AFC and World Sport Group (WSG) negotiated by Bin Hammam without putting it out to tender or financial due diligence.[10]

This writer's reporting on the audit led to a libel case in Singapore that he won in 2014 in a landmark ruling that changed Singapore court procedures and enhanced the right of appeal in libel cases.[11] The libel case fit a pattern of attempts by Salman and Prince Nasser bin Hamad Al Khalifa, a relative and Bahrain's sports czar, to halt this writer as well as others from writing critically about them by employing by high-powered London lawyers and threatening costly legal action. With the exception of the Singapore case, Salman and Nasser backed down when intimidation failed to halt critical reporting and analysis.

The AFC and Salman have, meanwhile, refused to act on the recommendations of the audit, let alone get to the bottom of the allegations. The only action they took was the firing of General Secretary Soosay in June 2015, after this writer disclosed a video that documented his attempts to undermine the PwC auditors by seeking to destroy documents. Officially, Soosay, who denied the allegations, resigned voluntarily. He has since been hired as a consultant.[12]

Mushrooming scandals

The AFC's ability to snub its nose at FIFA has had far-reaching consequences for global soccer governance, no more so since Bin Hammam became AFC president in 2002. Men like Bin Hammam, Salman, and Ahmad are imperious and ambitious, who worked assiduously to concentrate power in their own hands and sideline their critics clamouring for reform. Hailing from countries governed by absolutist, hereditary leaders, they have been accused of being willing to occupy their seats of power at whatever price with persistent allegations of bribery and vote buying in their electoral campaigns. Personal and national ambition, corruption and greed led to Bin Hammam's ultimate downfall. Bin Hammam was banned in 2012 for life from involvement in professional soccer for 'conflict of interest', a euphemism for improper financial management of the affairs of the AFC as well as of his role in the Qatari World Cup bid.[13]

FIFA's mushrooming scandals, culminating in the indictment in 2015 in the United States of senior FIFA executives and a joint raid on FIFA in Zurich by US and Swiss law enforcement officials as the group gathered for the election of a new president, and a Swiss investigation into the awarding of the Russia and Qatar World Cups in 2018 and 2022,[14] forced the organization to introduce reforms. Members of the old guard associated with the era of disgraced FIFA president Sepp Blatter who stepped down in 2016 have been expelled. FIFA's management structure was overhauled and scores of officials were penalized. Yet, the incestuous relationship between sports and politics remained untouched. 'Even if radical change is welcomed in world football politics, there is an increasing worry that the means to achieve this change might be as corrupted as it was under the old guard', noted Norwegian soccer journalist Pal Odegard.[15]

That suspicion is substantiated by the composition of global and regional soccer governance boards, FIFA's lack of sincerity in pushing Qatar to reform its controversial labour system that goes to the core of criticism of the World Cup awarding, and international soccer governance's burial of allegations that Salman and his former Bahraini superior and relative, Prince Nasser bin Hamad Al Khalifa were involved in the arrest and violations of human rights of scores of athletes and sports officials accused of having participated in mass anti-government protests in Bahrain in 2011. Both men have consistently denied any wrongdoing.[16] The suspicion is reinforced by the autocratic traits of men like Salman and Nasser reflected in their multiple attempts to squash investigative reporting through intimidation by highly paid lawyers.[17] It is also reflected in the AFC's failure to properly investigate financial and political mismanagement laid bare in the independent audit and follow-up on the audit's recommendations.[18]

FIFA in the walk-up to its 2015 presidential election, in which Salman was viewed as a frontrunner, requested information from the Bahrain Football Association (BFA) about the arrest and torture of the soccer players at a time that Salman was secretary general of the national Olympic committee presided by Nasser and head of the BFA. FIFA pressure persuaded Bahraini authorities to release two players, brothers Alaa and Mohammed Hubail, but refrained from properly investigating the BFA or holding it accountable. FIFA's committee charged with the investigation refused to consider incriminating statements published by Bahrain's state-owned, tightly controlled news agency that serves as the distributor of government news. At the same time, Salman employed lawyers on at least four occasions to unsuccessfully intimidate this author or media outlets that run his syndicated column.

The intertwining of sports and politics is prevalent in sports governance in the Middle East. Thirteen Middle Eastern national associations account for 28% of the AFC's 46 member associations. As a result, the composition of the AFC's executive committee speaks volumes. Seven of the AFC executive committee's 23 members hail from the Middle East. Two are members of ruling families, four have close ties to the regime of their countries and one is the deputy commander of the Abu Dhabi police and director of the UAE's National Emergency and Crisis Management Authority (NCEMA).

Salman is not the only Middle Eastern AFC executive whose associations raise human rights-related questions. The AFC referred questions about the CV of its executive committee member, Major General Mohammed Khalfan Al Romaithi, the police commander and former head of the UAE football association, to the UAE federation, which did not respond to email requests and was unreachable by phone.

Human Rights Watch researcher Nicholas McGeehan noted that 'with the police … there seems to be … more of a pattern of general mistreatment and abuse (Personal communication to the author, 4 April 2017)'.[19] The UK's Foreign & Commonwealth Office said in a letter in 2015 that it was aware of '43 cases of complaints by British nationals of torture or mistreatment within the justice system in the United Arab Emirates over the last five-year period'. Of these 43 cases, 37 relate to Dubai and six to Abu Dhabi.[20] One of those complainants was former Leeds United director David Haigh, who spent two years in detention in the UAE.

One particular brutal incident occurred in 2009 when a uniformed officer helped Sheikh Issa bin Zayed al Nahyan, a brother of the country's crown prince and deputy military commander, Sheikh Mohammed bin Zayed al-Nahyan, as well as Sheikh Mansour bin Zayed al-Nahyan, the owner of English premier club Manchester City tie a man with tape, torture him with whips, electric cattle prods and wooden planks with protruding nails, pour salt on his wounds and then hold him down as a Mercedes SUV drives over him.[21] Human rights organizations have since repeatedly taken the UAE to task for disappearing and abusing critics of the government.

The Middle Eastern pattern of close ties between sport and politics are further evident in Asia not only in the AFC but also in organizations like the Olympic Council of Asia (OCA). The Kuwait-based OCA is headed by Sheikh Ahmed, a former oil minister, who also presides the Association of National Olympic Committees (ANOC) and is believed to harbour political ambitions in his home country and to play a major behind-the-scenes role in AFC politics. Ahmad has manipulated the fiction of a separation between sports and politics to his advantage with the suspension of Kuwait by the IOC, FIFA, the AFC and most other international sports associations as a result of a political power struggle to which he is a key party.[22] The associations have accused Kuwait of political interference in the country's sports governance. Claiming that it was tackling financial irregularities, Kuwait in August 2016 dissolved the country's National Olympic Committee and soccer association in a bid to undermine Ahmad's power.[23]

Earlier, Kuwait's Public Authority for Youth and Sports headed by Sheikh Ahmad Mansour Al-Ahmad Al-Sabah, another relative of Sheikhs Ahmed, sued him as well as his brother, Sheikh Talal Fahad Ahmad J Al-Sabah, and other members of the NOC for $1.3 billion in damages. The authority asserted that the damages resulted from Sheikh Ahmad's complaint to the IOC about government interference. Youth Minister Sheikh Salman Sabah Al-Salem Al-Homud Al-Sabah charged without mentioning him by name that Sheikh Ahmed was responsible for the "total decline" in Kuwaiti sports. Sheikh Salman claimed that the decline stemmed from 'false complaints to international organizations in a bid to suspend the country's sport activities'.[24]

Founded in 1982, the OCA has only had two presidents, Ahmed since 1991, and his father and brother of Kuwait's ruler, Sheikh Fahad Al-Ahmad Al-Sabah (Olympic Council of Asia).[25] Of the OCA's 41 executive board members, 12 hail from the Middle East. Three of the Middle Easterners are Kuwaitis, including Ahmed's brother, Sheikh Talal Fahad Ahmad J Al-Sabah and two others (Olympic Council of Asia).[26] Three others are members of ruling families while two others, including a brigadier general in the military of embattled Syrian president Bashar al-Assad that stands accused of war crimes and a member of Syria's rubber stamp parliament, are military officers. Brigadier General Mowaffak Joumaa, who also serves as head of the Syrian Olympic committee in a country where the military controls sports associations and major clubs, was denied a visa to attend the 2012 London Olympics because of his close ties to Al-Assad.[27]

The pattern of political control of sports repeats itself in the Middle East at the level of the West Asian Football Federation (WAFF) that groups the region's associations except for Israel as well as at the level of national associations. At least half of the West Asian Football Federation's 13 members are headed by members of ruling families or people closely associated with them. This includes Kuwait, Oman, Bahrain, Qatar and Jordan.

Saudi Arabia's soccer association remains tightly controlled by the kingdom's General Presidency of Youth Welfare that is headed by a member of the ruling Al Saud family even after former Saudi Arabian Football Federation (SAFF) president, Prince Nawaf bin Faisal, became in 2012 the Gulf's first royal to resign under popular pressure. Members of the board of the Football Federation of the Islamic Republic of Iran (FFIRI) are closely linked to Iran's Army of the Guardians of the Islamic Revolution popularly known as Pasdaran or Revolutionary Guards while many of its clubs are owned by state entities. Similarly, clubs in the Gulf and Syria are frequently owned by members of ruling families and state institutions, including the military and security forces.

Qatar: the lightening rod

FIFA's double-barrelled awarding of hosting rights for the 2018 World Cup to Russia and the 2022 tournament to Qatar[28] put the group's incestuous relationship to politics as well as its marriage to Arab autocracy centre stage. The awarding fuelled already widespread suspicions of massive corruption of global soccer governance and the awarding process. Qatar or soccer officials who were either members of Gulf ruling families or close to them played key roles in scandals that ensued. Lurking in the shadows behind Bin Hammam in the controversy about the 2022 World Cup, was former Qatari Emir Sheikh Hamad Bin Khalifa Al Thani, and his son and current emir, Sheikh Tamim bin Hamad Al Than, who Bin Hammam knew from childhood.

Already a member of FIFA's executive committee and head of the AFC, Bin Hammam gunned for the FIFA presidency within months of securing Qatar's World Cup hosting rights. Bin Hammam was a formidable challenger to Blatter, who was seeking a fourth term.[29] In preventing Bin Hammam to stand in the May 2011 FIFA presidential election, Blatter exploited Bin Hammam's Achilles Heel: a failure to realize that while standards of business in the Gulf and in FIFA were similar, FIFA could apply the Western rules governing conflict of interest and bribery whenever it wished. Bin Hammam was banned for life in 2013 for having violated FIFA rules on conflict of interest.[30]

Blatter was aided in his defeat of Bin Hammam by a Qatari realization that gaining leadership of FIFA with controversy over the Gulf state's hosting of the World Cup would likely complicate rather than advance its effort to enhance Qatari soft power through sports. It was also Gulf politics that stopped Bin Hammam, convinced of his innocence, from further fighting the FIFA ban. Sheikh Tamim, the Qatari emir, stopped Bin Hamam as part of a deal with Blatter to ensure that Qatar would not lose its hosting rights.[31]

Politics is also what reduces FIFA reform to a formality. The soccer body went through the motions when it established in 2016 a watchdog to monitor the living and working conditions of migrant labour employed on World Cup 2022-related construction sites. The long-overdue FIFA move more than five years after Qatar was awarded World Cup hosting rights constituted the first concrete follow-up to a report by Harvard University international affairs and human rights professor John Ruggie, a renowned human rights scholar, that called on FIFA to 'consider suspending or terminating' its relationship with World Cup hosts who fail to clean up their human rights records. The watchdog has yet to take any substantial actions or make any statements of substance.[32]

For FIFA, it was a missed opportunity to polish its tarnished image by capitalizing on the fact that with the adoption of Ruggie's report on FIFA it became the first international sports federation to formally make human rights an integral part of its processes, procedures and decisions. The guidelines, according to Ruggie, would oblige FIFA to 'apply maximum leverage' to address existing human rights issues and 'to withdraw from contracts' if its efforts fail (Personal communication to the author, 14 December 2015).[33]

A balancing act

The balancing act that international sports associations perform in their relations to Middle East autocracies and theocracies is particularly acute when it comes to the ban of women to attend male sporting events in Iran and Saudi Arabia.

> It's humiliating. First you belong to your father and brother, then to your husband and son who can do with you what they want. It is humiliating. How can you say that women's rights go against culture? The problem is: who cares about women's rights?

said Darya Safai, a 41-year-old Iranian student activist-turned dentist and women's sports campaigner who was jailed in Iran before fleeing via Turkey to Belgium (Personal communication to the author, 15 March 2014).[34]

Safai, who travels the world to sporting mega events at which she unfolds a banner demanding women's unfettered access to stadiums in Iran, sees her activism rooted in her first encounters as a child with discrimination of women. In line with Iranian dress code, her mother forced her at age six on her first day of school to exchange the clothes she liked for a body enveloping blue mantle and a head cover. 'I realized something was wrong when I saw my neighbour's son going to school in the same clothes he always wore. Nothing had changed for him. From that moment on, I wanted to be a boy', Safai said.

Safai was subsequently admonished by teachers for laughing out loud because that was improper.

> I was afraid in school. I look at pictures from that time and I'm never smiling because girls aren't supposed to display their teeth. From age nine, we were taught that you would go to hell if a man sees you. I was afraid of the pain of burning in hell. Later my bicycle was taken from me. It was terrorizing children … At a given moment, the penny dropped. I realized it's not my fault. That was my rebellion. I wanted my rights,

she said speaking fluent Dutch in an Antwerp café.

Safai had a taste of those rights in 1997, when thousands of Iranian male and female soccer fans poured into the streets of Tehran to celebrate Iran's defeat of Australia with a last-minute goal in a World Cup qualifier that paved the way for the Islamic Republic's joining the 1998 World Cup finals. 'It was a day on which everything that was forbidden became possible. Men and women were on the streets. The veils were off, they danced and sang together. It was one of the most beautiful days of my life', Safai recalls.

Two thousand twelve was a watershed in Safai's struggle for women's sporting rights in the Middle East in several ways. It was the year in which FIFA and the International Football Association Board (IFAB) that sets the rules of the game opened the door to religiously observant Muslim women to play in international competitions with their hair covered.[35] WAFF adopted months later a resolution that put the right of a woman to compete on par with that of a man. Eleven of the federation's 13 member associations, including Iran, voted in favour. Saudi Arabia, which like Iran bans women from attending men's sports competitions, and Yemen voted against. The resolution was revolutionary even if it only had symbolic value because the federation didn't have the teeth to enforce it.[36]

Two thousand twelve was also the year in which the International Olympic Committee (IOC) prompted by the head of its Women and Sports Commission for the first time threatened the world's three countries – Saudi Arabia, Qatar and Brunei – that had never sent a woman to an Olympic sporting event, with a boycott if women were not included in their representations in London.[37] Saudi Arabia avoided a boycott by sending two expatriate athletes. What has evolved since in both the case of Saudi Arabia and Iran is a cat and mouse game in which international sports associations effectively have thrown the towel into the ring in effect allowing the two countries to maintain misogynist policies. Pressure since by the IOC to force Saudi Arabia to take necessary measures to institutionalize women's sports, including introduction of mandatory sports lessons in girl's schools, development of an infrastructure that would foster women's elite sports, and adoption of policies to encourage and enable female participation, have lacked the resolve necessary to produce results that went beyond the kingdom doubling its women delegate to four at the 2016 Rio Olympics.

Iran, however, has proven slightly more receptive. Bowing to external pressure, Iran in early 2017, allowed women spectators to attend a premier international men's volleyball tournament on the island of Kish. The Iranian concession constituted a rare occasion on which the Islamic republic has not backtracked on promises to international sports associations to lift its ban on women attending men's sporting events. Human rights groups hailed the move as a positive, albeit small step forward.[38]

The Iranian concession followed a decision by the Federation Internationale de Volleyball (FIVB) to dump its quiet diplomacy approach towards Iran and revert to public pressure. The FIVB threatened on the eve of the Kish tournament to suspend the event if Iran failed to grant female spectators access.[39] 'From now on women can watch beach volleyball matches in Kish if they observe Islamic rules', said Kasra Ghafouri, acting director of Iran's Beach Volleyball Organisation forward.[40]

The FIVB has flip-flopped in its attitude towards Iran. The group initially took a lead among international sports associations in publicly declaring that it would not grant Iran hosting rights if women were not given unfettered access to stadia. In response, Iran promised to allow women to attend international volleyball tournaments in the Islamic republic. Taking Iranian authorities by their word, women travelled last year to Kish for the 2016 tournament only to discover that Iran would not make good on its promise.

Rather than demonstrating sincerity by following through on its threat, the FIVB said it would not sanction the Islamic republic because gender segregation was culturally so deep-seated that a boycott would not produce results. Instead, the federation argued that engagement held out more promise. The decision flew in the face of the facts. Gender segregation in volleyball in Iran was only introduced in 2012, 33 years after Islamic revolutionaries toppled the Shah. Senior volleyball executives said at the time that the FIVB feared that a boycott would put significant revenues at risk[41]

Conclusion

What these scandals, crises and controversies have in common is far more than a coincidental involvement of Gulf personalities. They all reflect in extremity the problems involved in the relationship between sports and politics, an inseparable and incestuous relationship that is allowed to flourish unregulated and ungoverned with international sports associations and governments misleadingly denying that the relationship even exists. The fiction of a separation of politics and sports not only impacts the integrity of governance but as in the case of women the rights of segments of society. The beneficiaries are autocrats and bureaucrats who have a vested interest in the status quo. They both are well served by upholding the fiction of a separation of politics and sports. Theirs is a mutually beneficial marriage made in heaven.

Notes

1. Future for Advanced Research and Studies, The Political Dimension of Sports in the Middle East, Email to the author, 19 February 2017.
2. Dorsey, James M. 2017. "Middle East Soccer: Trump's Israel-Palestine Peace Making Put to the Test." The Turbulent World of Middle East Soccer, March 24. https://mideastsoccer.blogspot.co.uk/2017/03/middle-east-soccer-trumps-israel.html.

3. Houlihan, Barrie. 2000. "Politics and Sports." In *Handbook of Sports Studies*, edited by Jay Coakley and Eric Dunning, 218. London: Sage / Little, Charles. 2012. "Asia, South and East." In *Sports Around the World, History, Culture and Practice*. Vol. 1, edited by John Nauright and Charles Parrish, 186. Santa Barbara: ABC-CLIO.

4. Article 3 of the FIFA as well as the AFC Statutes states: 'Discrimination of any kind against a country, private person or group of people on account of ethnic origin, gender, language, religion, politics or any other reason is strictly prohibited and punishable by suspension or expulsion'. http://www.fifa.com/mm/document/affederation/generic/01/09/75/14/fifa_statutes_072008_en.pdf/http://www.the-waff.com/assets/files/78_3_1387199813.pdf.

5. Agence France Presse. 2015. "Football: AFC 'Broad-minded' on Iranian Women Ban." *The Times of India*, January 23. http://timesofindia.indiatimes.com/sports/football/top-stories/.

6. Velappan, Peter. 2014. *Beyond Dreams, The Fascinating Story of The Blessed Life of Peter Velappan*. Kuala Lumpur: Peter Velappan s/o Palaniappan.

7. Dorsey, James M. 2016. *The Turbulent World of Middle East Soccer*. London/New York: Hurst/Oxford University Press.

8. Salomon, Patrick. 2008. "Shaikh Salman FIFA Bid Backed." *Gulf Daily News*. http://www.gulf-daily-news.com/Print.aspx?storyid=245608.

9. Dorsey, James M. 2016. "Bahraini's Soccer Defeat: A Cautionary Tale for Autocrats." *The Turbulent World of Middle East Soccer*, February 27. https://mideastsoccer.blogspot.co.uk/2016/02/bahrainis-soccer-defeat-cautionary-tale.html.

10. Dorsey, James M. 2012. "Bin Hammam Audit Opens Pandora's Box." *The Turbulent World of Middle East Soccer*, July 23. http://mideastsoccer.blogspot.sg/2012/07/bin-hammam-audit-opens-pandoras-box.html.

11. SingaporeLaw. 2014. *Dorsey James Michael v World Sport Group Pte Ltd*. SGCA 4, January 14. http://www.singaporelaw.sg/sglaw/laws-of-singapore/case-law/free-law/court-of-appeal-judgments/15485-dorsey-james-michael-v-world-sport-group-pte-ltd-2014-sgca-4.

12. Dorsey, James M. 2016. "AFC Rehires Former Executive Accused of Seeking to Destroy Corruption-related Documents." *The Turbulent World of Middle East Soccer*, March 30. https://mideastsoccer.blogspot.co.uk/2016/03/afc-rehires-former-executive-accused-of.html.

13. Dorsey, James M. 2012. "Bin Hammam Banning Puts AFC Marketing Contract in the Firing Line." *The Turbulent World of Middle East Soccer*, December 18. https://mideastsoccer.blogspot.co.uk/2012/12/bin-hammam-banning-puts-afc-marketing.html.

14. Dorsey, James M. 2015. "Qatar's Unintended Sporting Legacy: A FIFA Clean-up, Exposure of Political Corruption, and Corporate Sponsor Rethink." *The Turbulent World of Middle East Soccer*, May 28. https://mideastsoccer.blogspot.co.uk/2015/05/qatars-unintended-sporting-legacy-fifa.html.

15. Odegard, Pal. 2017. "Infantino's African Victory." *Josimar*, March 25. http://www.josimar.no/artikler/infantinos-african-victory/3837/?utm_content=bufferb191f&utm_medium=social&utm_source=twitter.com&utm_campaign=buffer.

16. Dorsey, James M. 2016. Salman's Moral Rectitude or Everything You Wanted to Know About FIFA But Never Dared to Ask." *The Turbulent World of Middle East Soccer*, February 21. http://mideastsoccer.blogspot.com/2016/02/salmans-moral-rectitude-or-everything.html.

17. Dorsey, James M. 2016. "Pressure Builds on Sheikh Salman to Respond to Human Rights Allegations." *The Turbulent World of Middle East Soccer*, January 20. https://mideastsoccer.blogspot.co.uk/2016/01/pressure-builds-on-sheikh-salman-to.html.

18. Dorsey, James M. 2016. "AFC Rehires Former Executive Accused of Seeking to Destroy Corruption-related Documents." *The Turbulent World of Middle East Soccer*, March 16. https://mideastsoccer.blogspot.co.uk/2016/03/afc-rehires-former-executive-accused-of.html.

19. Email to the author, 4 April 2017.

20. Consular Directorate, Letter to Alison Fong San Pin of Lawrence & Co. Solicitors, Foreign & Commonwealth Office, 29 June 2015.

21. El Buri, Vic Walter Rehab, Angela Hill, and Brian Ross. 2009. "ABC News Exclusive: Torture Tape Implicates UAE Royal Sheikh." *ABC News*, April 22. http://abcnews.go.com/Blotter/story?id=7402099.

22. Dorsey, James M. 2016. "Kuwaiti Rulers Fight Their Internal Battles on the Sports Field." *The Turbulent World of Middle East Soccer*, June 19. http://mideastsoccer.blogspot.com/2016/06/kuwaiti-rulers-fight-their-internal.html.
23. Wickstrom, Mads A. 2016. "Kuwait Dissolves Olympic Committee and National Football Association." *Play the Game*, 29 August. http://www.playthegame.org/news/news-articles/2016/0219_kuwait-dissolves-olympic-committee-and-national-football-association/.
24. Ibid. Dorsey, Kuwaiti rulers.
25. Olympic Council of Asia, Presidents, http://www.ocasia.org/council/President.aspx.
26. Olympic Council of Asia, OCA Executive Board Members – Current Members, http://www.ocasia.org/council/ExeBoard.aspx.
27. Magnay, Jacquelin. 2012. "London 2012 Olympics: Syria's Games Chief General Mowaffak Joumaa is Banned But Athletes Will Compete." *The Telegraph*, June 22. http://www.telegraph.co.uk/sport/olympics/9349019/London-2012-Olympics-Syrias-Games-chief-General-Mowaffak-Joumaa-is-banned-but-athletes-will-compete.html.
28. FIFA. 2010. *Russia and Qatar awarded 2018 and 2022 FIFA World Cups*, December 2. http://www.fifa.com/worldcup/news/y=2010/m=12/news=russia-and-qatar-awarded-2018-and-2022-fifa-world-cups-1344698.html.
29. Dorsey, James M. 2011. "FIFA Temporarily Bans Bin Hammam But Clears Blatter of Corruption Charges." *The Turbulent World of Middle East Soccer*, May 30. https://mideastsoccer.blogspot.co.uk/2011/05/fifa-temporarily-bans-bin-hammam-but.html.
30. FIFA. 2012. *Mohamed Bin Hammam Resigns from Football, Banned for Life*, December 17. http://www.fifa.com/governance/news/y=2012/m=12/news=mohamed-bin-hammam-resigns-from-football-banned-for-life-1973422.html.
31. Blake, Heidi and Jonathan Calvert. 2015. *The Ugly Game: The Corruption of FIFA and the Qatari Plot to Buy the World Cup*. Kindle edition. New York: Scribner.
32. Dorsey, James M. 2016. "FIFA, Human Rights and Politics: One Step Forward, Two Steps Backwards." *The Turbulent World of Middle East Soccer*, April 23. https://mideastsoccer.blogspot.co.uk/2016/04/fifa-human-rights-and-politics-one-step.html.
33. Interview with the author, 14 December 2015.
34. Interview with the author, 15 March 2014.
35. Nkeuna, Frédéric. 2014. "World Cup is Next Goal for Soccer Teens in Hijab." *We News*, April 11. http://womensenews.org/2014/04/world-cup-next-goal-soccer-teens-in-hijab/.
36. Dorsey, James M. 2013. "Middle East Soccer Associations Campaign for Women's Right to Play." *The Turbulent World of Middle East Soccer*, January 14, https://mideastsoccer.blogspot.co.uk/2013/01/middle-east-soccer-associations.html.
37. *BBC News*. 2012. "London 2012 Olympics: Saudi Arabian Women to Compete," July 12. http://www.bbc.com/news/world-middle-east-18813543.
38. *Human Rights Watch*. 2017. "Iran: Women Allowed to Attend Kish Island Open," February 17. https://www.hrw.org/news/2017/02/17/iran-women-allowed-attend-kish-island-open.
39. *Associated Press*. 2015. "Iran Allows Female Spectators at Beach Volleyball Tournament," February 15. https://apnews.com/ba007817d4624c038cf27e299db8ea83/Iran-allows-female-spectators-at-beach-volleyball-tournament?utm_campaign=SocialFlow&utm_source=Twitter&utm_medium=AP_Sports.
40. Ibid. Human Rights Watch.
41. Dorsey, James M. 2017. "Bowing to Pressure: Iran Grants Women Spectators Access to Sporting Event," *The Turbulent World of Middle East Soccer*, February 19. https://mideastsoccer.blogspot.sg/2017/02/bowing-to-pressure-iran-grants-women.html.

Disclosure statement

No potential conflict of interest was reported by the author.

Towards responsible policy-making in international sport: reforming the medical-scientific commissions

Bruce Kidd[#]

ABSTRACT

On 24 July 2015, the Court of Arbitration for Sport upheld an appeal by Indian sprinter Dutee Chand against the Hyperandrogenism Regulations of the International Association of Athletics Federations (IAAF), finding that the IAAF could not provide sufficient scientific evidence to justify the Regulations. It was the first time that CAS had overturned both an athlete's suspension and the relevant policy. The decision should have prompted the IAAF and the International Olympic Committee, which had similar regulations, to re-examine the processes by which they have imposed their rules upon the female athletes of the world, but both bodies hunkered down and defended the suspended policies. This paper argues that the IAAF and the IOC established the hyperandrogenism regulations in a conspiratorial, unsubstantiated and harmful manner that flies in the face of the 'best practice' established by other bodies that create science-based policies affecting large numbers of people and tarnishes the Olympic Movement. I call upon the IAAF and IOC to reform the medical commissions by requiring future policy-making along the lines of the guidelines established by international organizations such as the World Health Organization.

Introduction

On 24 July 2015, the Court of Arbitration for Sport (CAS) upheld the appeal by Indian sprinter Dutee Chand against the International Association of Athletics Federation's (IAAF) 'Regulations Governing the Eligibility of Females to Compete in Women's Competition' (the Hyperandrogenism Regulations) (CAS 2015). The Regulations had stipulated that female athletes with naturally elevated testosterone levels were to be suspended or banned outright unless they underwent medical intervention to lower their testosterone levels. A year previously, on 13 July 2014, on the eve of her anticipated participation in the Commonwealth Games in Glasgow, Chand had been suddenly barred from competition on the grounds that her natural testosterone levels were too high and that she had violated the Regulations. When her suspension was leaked to the media, the Kolkata-based social

[#]I am extremely grateful for the insights and advice of Lisa Davington, James Bunting, Michele Donnelly, Peter Donnelly, Katrina Karkazis, Payoshni Mitra and Carlos Sayao and the courageous examples of Dutee Chand and Caster Semanya. The views expressed in this paper and any errors or omissions, however, are completely my own.

scientist Payoshni Mitra contacted Chand, who asked for help in challenging her suspension. Mitra recruited Katrina Karkazis and the author as advisors, the Sport Authority of India to provide financial, administrative and communications support and the Toronto-based legal team of James Bunting and Carlos Sayao to conduct the appeal on a pro bono basis (Gillespie 2016a; Nolen 2016; Slater 2015). Chand filed her formal appeal with CAS on 26 September 2014.

It was an historic decision by the Lausanne-based 'supreme court' of international sport. In its carefully worded 162-page judgement, the three-person presiding panel (chaired by the Hon. Annabelle Claire Bennett of the Federal Court of Australia with arbitrators Richard McLaren of Canada and Hans Nater of Switzerland) unconditionally restored Chand to competition. It also suspended the very policy on which her ban was based for two years, or until such time within that two-year period that the IAAF could persuade CAS that there is compelling scientific evidence to demonstrate that naturally high testosterone levels actually give hyperandrogenic female athletes an unfair advantage as compared to their peers. If the IAAF could not convincingly make the case for the Regulations, the panel ruled, the Regulations would be forever null and void. It was the first time in its 31-year history that CAS had overturned an athlete's suspension *and* the relevant policy. Since the IAAF Regulations were similar to those of the International Olympic Committee (IOC) for all the Olympic sports, the ruling removed the burden of the hyperandrogenism requirement and the accompanying scrutiny from every woman preparing for the 2016 Olympics in Rio.

In its decision, CAS determined that the IAAF had not provided sufficient scientific evidence to justify such actions:

> The IAAF has not discharged its onus of establishing that the Hyperandrogenism Regulations are necessary and proportionate to pursue the legitimate objective of organising competitive female athletics to ensure fairness in athletic competition. Specifically, the IAAF has not provided sufficient scientific evidence about the quantitative relationship between enhanced testosterone levels and improved athletic performance in hyperandrogenic athletes. In the absence of such evidence, the Panel is unable to conclude that hyperandrogenic female athletes may enjoy such a significant performance advantage that it is necessary to exclude them from competing in the female category. (CAS, para 547, 158)

The verdict laid bare what critics of the medical and scientific policies of the IOC and the international federations have been arguing for years (e.g. Bavington 2016; Canada 1991; Ferguson-Smith and Ferris 1991; Karkazis et al. 2012), namely that such policies have been initiated, approved and implemented with very little of the scientific rigour, critical peer review, consultation with those affected and concern for human rights that one would expect from governing bodies whose rules significantly affect large numbers of people around the world. The decision should have been a wake-up call to the IAAF and IOC that the processes by which their policies have been developed and promulgated are wholly inadequate to the needs of fair sport and should be significantly reformed. Yet the governing bodies dug in to defend the status quo. The IOC kept the world waiting six months before acknowledging that the CAS ruling applied to all Olympic federations and confirming that the Hyperandrogenism Regulations would not be applied to those athletes preparing for the 2016 Olympic Games in Rio de Janeiro (Gillespie 2016b). That delay caused considerable anxiety among athletes in many countries (Mitra 2015). In January 2016, the IOC Medical and Scientific Commission reiterated its support of the Regulations and urged the IAAF to 'revert to CAS with arguments and evidence to support the reinstatement of its hyperandrogenism rules' (IOC 2016). During the Rio Games, IAAF President Sebastian Coe announced that the athletics body would mount a formal challenge to the CAS decision, (*Guardian* 11 August 2016). It then waited until the very last month of the two-year window, until 4 July 2017, before formally indicating that it would actually do so, in India, on the eve of the Indian national championships where Chand was racing the very next day. The announcement only reignited the anxiety among athletes and the broad support Chand enjoys among the Indian public and many others in the world (Press Trust of India 2017).

The arguments (and counter-arguments by Chand and her legal team) will focus on the bar set by CAS, namely is there sufficient scientific evidence to justify the Regulations. This would appear to be an impossible task. The research (Bermon 2017; Bermon and Garnier 2017) cited by the IAAF in its announcement of the challenge, led by IAAF and IOC medical commission member Stéphane Bermon and financially supported by the IAAF and the World Anti-Doping Agency, offers no new evidence to suggest that the IAAF could overturn the original decision. After studying 2127 competitors at the 2011 and 2013 athletics world championships, Bermon and Garnier argue that women with high natural testosterone levels in some events (but not others) enjoyed between a 1.78 and a 4.53% advantage over women whose natural testosterone falls within the 'normal' range. That is little changed from the 1–3% advantage Bermon argued at CAS. The CAS panel suggested that the advantage would have to be in the 12% range to consider a policy of differentiation (CAS 532–534, 154, 155; see also the criticism of Bermon and Garnier's analysis by Karkazis and Meyerowitz-Katz 2017).

Why did the IAAF and IOC get it so wrong? Many others have exposed the Western, patriarchal biases and faulty logic of the authors of the Hyperandrogenism Regulations (e.g. Henne 2014; Karkazis and Jordan-Young 2013; Padawer 2016; Pieper 2014; Schultz 2011). In this paper, I critique the process by which the IAAF and IOC established the Hyperandrogenism Regulations and applied them to female athletes around the world. In both cases, the Regulations were recommended by standing 'commissions' appointed for medical and health related matters, the 'Medical and Anti-Doping Commission' in the case of the IAAF and the 'Medical and Scientific Commission' in the case of the IOC, and then confirmed by their respective governing bodies. These commissions have much to be proud of but, I will argue, the Hyperandrogenism Regulations were initiated and implemented in a conspiratorial, unsubstantiated and harmful manner that flies in the face of the 'best practice' established by other bodies that create science-based policies affecting large numbers of people. Although the IOC has introduced many welcome reforms to its governance processes during the last few decades, especially those initiated by the 2000 Commission appointed by President Samaranch and Olympic Agenda 2020 appointed by President Bach, the way the medical commissions operate has escaped this attention.

Sports bodies assume enormous power over an essential sphere of everyday life and the individuals and institutions who participate in the activities they govern. The rules they establish – and the way those rules are implemented – can transform the lives of athletes and entire communities. The Hyperandrogenism Regulations were particularly harsh and severe: they stipulated that female athletes whose natural biochemistry did not meet their standards were to be suspended from sport for life, unless those athletes agreed to undergo hormonal therapy or surgery. This latter possibility was not hypothetical: in the first three years of the Regulations, four cases of irreversible surgery were documented in otherwise healthy women (Fénichal et al. 2013; cf. Sonksen et al. 2015; United Nations 2016). Because the test could be triggered by appearance or an official's look, the Regulations created enormous stress among women, if not a body-image chill for every woman in the world. In her testimony before CAS, Katrina Karkazis argued that 'more than half the indicators specified in the Hyperandrogenism Regulations to determine which female athletes should undergo investigation are entangled with deeply subjective and stereotypically definitions of femininity' (CAS, 255, 76.) From the known tests, it has been only women from the Global South who have been singled out, suggesting a global system of racial profiling.

With the explosive expansion of the social media, the communication of sport decisions, especially prohibitions from competition, has implications far beyond the confines of sports – they provide symbolic examples for everyday debates about social policy in a wide range of fields. In virtually every country in the world, the sport bodies' power is enabled, provided and financed by governments and public institutions and is exercised in the public realm. For all these reasons, sports policies ought to meet the highest standards of public transparency and accountability. Yet in their regulations affecting the eligibility, health and well-being of athletes, international sports bodies have acted as if they do not need to be accountable to anyone, claiming the 'autonomy of sport'. If international sport is to continue to enjoy public confidence, the 'anatomy of sport' must be responsible, transparent, respectful of national and international law and internationally consistent.

The lesson of Dutee Chand is that a significant reform of the policy-making powers of the medical commissions of international sport is urgently required. I will recommend that in the creation of future policies, the medical commissions should institute multi-disciplinary peer-review, high standards of evidence, rules for conflict of interest, an open-nomination process for decision-makers, an open consultation process, including consultation with athletes and human rights experts, and arms-length decision-making for policies, and should plan for inclusive communication and education prior to implementation. I suggest that the World Health Organization's *Handbook for Guideline Development* is a good place to start. The IOC, IAAF and other international federations should insist upon these safeguards before even considering new policies. In the case of policies that solely affect women, the recommending body should be the IOC Women's Commission and the Athletes' Commission (and similar bodies in the international federations) not the medical and scientific commissions. My perspective is that of a lifelong participant in the Olympic Movement and an analyst and advisor on Canadian and international sports policy who has been deeply troubled by the persistent insensitivity of the Olympic leadership on this issue.

The medical commissions

The medical commissions were a product of the 1960s and 1970s. The IOC Medical Commission was established in 1961 in response to the tragic death of Danish cyclist Knud Jensen during the 100 km team time trial at the Rome Olympics. It took several years for the Commission to become fully operational, but by the late 1960s, it had assumed oversight for the medical facilities at Olympic and Winter Olympic Game and responsibility for 'doping control' and 'femininity control'. The IAAF Medical Committee was formed in 1972 with a similar mandate. In subsequent years, other international federations followed suit

(Beckett 1976; Chappelet and Kubler-Mabbott 2008; IAAF n.d.). Today the IOC's medical and scientific commission states its responsibilities as the 'protection of the health of athletes, respect for both medical and sports ethics, and equality for all competing athletes'. The IAAF medical and anti-doping commission focuses on the prevention of doping and the advance of sports medicine. There is much to commend in the work of the medical commissions, especially in the initiation of the fight against doping, the education and leadership development of coaches and officials and the encouragement and dissemination of research. The IOC's commission contributes to courses on sports medicine conducted by Olympic Solidarity; in 2015, 51 National Olympic Committees benefitted from such training (IOC 2015, 34). It publishes articles and books on issues related to athletes' health, including the multi-volume the *Encylopedia and Handbooks of Sports Medicine*, and now partners with a network of nine research centres around the world on the prevention of injury and the promotion of athletes' health. From time to time, it issues voluntary 'guidelines regarding the medical care and health of the athletes' (IOC n.d.) The IAAF's commission has conducted an injury surveillance programme at major competitions, with a view to prevent injury, and publishes advice on related topics, including nutrition and fluid replacement. The medical commission of the Fédération Internationale de Natation (the international federation for swimming) organizes an international congress every four years to review the latest sports science related to aquatics performance and health. Most of the work of the medical commissions work is carried out by volunteers.

But the track record of the medical commissions in the policy area has been mixed. Take doping. On the one hand, the medical commissions initiated and for many years led the fight against doping at the international level. The IOC commission conducted the very first anti-doping tests (at the 1968 Winter Olympic and Olympic Games) and up until the creation of the World Anti-Doping Agency (WADA), prepared and revised the list of banned substances, developed and conducted the appropriate detection methodologies, accredited the testing laboratories and established the system of penalties and disciplinary tribunals. On the other hand, it had neither the expertise nor capacity nor temperament adequately to deal with the complex scientific, ethical and legal issues arising from the system it imposed on the world. It struggled to keep abreast of the ever more sophisticated doping techniques and new pharmaceutical products. It made little effort to address the mounting costs of prohibition and policing, especially in the Global South where many sports bodies face enormous financial challenges. It rejected out of hand strategies such as harm reduction that critics suggest would be more health-focused, less contradictory to the ethic of high performance sport and less expensive. Decisions were increasingly vulnerable to the charge that the members of the medical commission were compromised by their relationships with the testing labs and the IOC. In large part in response to its blind spot to athletes' rights and natural justice, a growing number of incriminated athletes was successful in appealing their positive tests and associated penalties in civil court. Moreover, the IOC was unable to impose a unified system upon the international federations, so that policies and practices varied from sport to sport. By the late 1990s, it seemed that the IOC could or would do nothing to curtail the rapidly increasing use of performance-enhancing drugs, while the explosive Salt Lake City bribery scandal undermined the credibility of the IOC as a whole. In this context, governments began to take action of their own, creating national anti-doping policies and regulatory bodies and forging international agreements, such as the 10-country International Anti-Doping Arrangement forged in 1995. In 1999, amid widespread public consternation about the seeming epidemic in doping, the World Anti-Doping Conference recommended the creation of an independent international agency, what is now the World Anti-Doping Agency. With the adoption of the WADA Code in 2003, the IOC medical and scientific commission was reduced to overseeing the implementation of the Code at the time of Winter Olympic and Olympic Games.

The tortuous history of 'femininity control' not only illustrates the inadequacy of the medical commissions as regulatory bodies but the harm they create. From the very beginnings of female competition within the Coubertin Olympic Movement, the largely male governing bodies of the IOC, IAAF and other international federations have sought to control and place limits upon women's competition, by restricting the number and difficulty of sports and events in which women compete and policing women's eligibility (Donnelly and Donnelly 2013; Lenskyj 2013). In the latter case, this has meant questioning the eligibility of those women whose appearance did not conform to the conventional body-type of upper class Western societies and whose performances surpassed officials' expectations, what IOC policy-makers have always referred to as 'abnormal women'. While the authorities have justified the need for testing on the grounds of fair competition, arguing that female athletes who are too fast or too strong might not be women after all, decades of feminist scholarship suggests a more patriarchal objective, namely to limit the legitimacy and rewards women derive from success in the traditionally male preserve of sports. They point out that no competitor in the history of the test has been outed as a man masquerading as a woman and that modern sports continue to be organized and promoted as an explicit vehicle for strengthened masculinity and male power, so that breakthrough female athletes constitute a symbolic threat to that power and privilege. They also argue that such tests constitute a double-standard, as outliers in men's sport, with 'abnormal' characteristics such as exceptional height, reach and genetic make-up predominant in virtually every sport, yet are never screened out for these advantages (e.g. Cole 2000; Ritchie 2003).

The first sex testing in conjunction with the Olympics was undertaken quietly on the eve of the 1936 Games in Berlin on a few prominent athletes, such as American Helen Stephens. Following the Second World War, the IAAF and IOC began to require *all* female athletes to submit medical certificates for purposes of eligibility. These requirements were tightened in the 1960s when a universal test was introduced at every major games. The backdrop was the striking success of two new groups of 'abnormal women' – muscular Soviet-bloc athletes at a time when sport was increasingly becoming a symbolic battlefield in the cold war, and the 'different' looking female athletes from the newly independent nations of Africa, Asia and the Caribbean. In 1965, the IAAF ruled that 'all female competitors in the Olympic Games, Area Games and Area Championships appear before a medical panel who will be required to certify that they are qualified to compete in such events'. At the 1966 Commonwealth Games in Kingston, Jamaica, the first such games held in the Global South, and at the European Track and Field Championships later that year, all female athletes were required to undergo a physical examination by gynecologists. In 1968, the IOC modified the screen to the less intrusive chromosome smear (a small cell sample was taken from the tongue to analyse chromosomal composition) for all female athletes. The test created enormous stress for female competitors at an already stressful time. For those women who 'failed' the test, public humiliation ensured (Patino 2005). It quickly became apparent that the test was unreliable as either a measure of biological status or competitive advantage; one complication was that the results could vary for the same individual in different tests at different times.

Yet it took years of criticism from medical specialists, athletes and governments before the IAAF abolished the test in 1992 and the IOC (a slightly revised test) in 1999. Both bodies retained the option of further testing 'should suspicions arise'.

Such a 'suspicion' came with the victory of the South African Caster Semanya in the 800 metres at the 2009 World Athletics Championships in Berlin. Instead of congratulating her, several of her competitors and some coaches and journalists from Western countries accused her as being 'too masculine'. The IAAF succumbed to the moral panic and ordered Semanya to undergo testosterone testing. At the same time, the IOC directed National Olympic Committees (NOCs) to 'actively investigate any perceived deviation in sex characteristics'. In April 2011, the IAAF issued the now suspended Hyperandrogenism Regulations and on the eve of the 2012 Olympics in London, the IOC issued Regulations on Female Hyperandrogenism modelled on the IAAF rules. In the three years that followed, approximately 30 women were suspended for 'failing' the test, and counselled either to retire from the sport or undergo 'corrective' hormonal therapy or surgery. Despite requirement of confidentiality, the names of some of those athletes have been revealed, subjecting those women to community isolation, if not humiliation and danger. All of those who have been publicly identified live and train in the Global South. It was Chand's courageous refusal of medical intervention, and her determination to overturn the Regulations that led to the CAS decision.

Given the reach of the Regulations – all female athletes in the world – the seriousness of the consequences of a failed test and the Olympic Movement's commitment to human rights, one would have expected a transparent, evidence-based, peer-reviewed and openly consultative approach to the development and approval of such a policy, and a rights-sensitive, educationally focused, strategy of implementation. Such was never the case:

Decisions made in secret, narrowly recruited meetings

The recommendation to create new regulations came from a by-invitation-only secret meeting – the IOC's Gender in Sport Symposium, held on 17–18 January 2010 in Miami, USA – without any outside consultation or opportunity for review. While the secret meeting was reported in the New York Times (Kolata 2010), no invitation list or formal recommendation was ever made public. What is particularly disconcerting is that the meeting in question was held immediately following a scientific meeting on the 'biological, genetic and psychological differences between the sexes' and the need to clarify 'problems of assigning sexual identification and managing those with atypical presentations', the very topics that the IOC Symposium would consider, in the very same Miami facility. Although the 2nd World Congress on the Hormonal and Genetic Basis of Sex Differentiation and Hot Topics in Endocrinology on 15–17 January was open to all scientists and scholars, the Symposium was closed. As the Proceedings show, the Congress heard wide-ranging discussions about the issues related to gender verification and hyperandrogenism, but no clear agreement on either the analysis or the policy options (New and Simpson 2011). Cassandra Wells, one of the Congress participants who was not invited to the IOC meeting, observed:

> Without a clear consensus regarding a proper approach to gender verification, the conference concluded and the selected experts retired to their next set of deliberations, this time with IOC officials. The outcome … reported an apparent agreement among the advisors on the recommended approach for the IOC. While this approach certainly echoed some of the (positions

stated in the open conference), it also contradicted many others', and failed to account for the experiences of those who were directed through the (recommended) approach and came out rejecting it. (Wells 2010)

A final by-invitation-only meeting was held in Lausanne in October 2010. It was the decisions of these meetings that led to the adoption of the IAAF policy on hyperandrogenism in 2011 and the IOC policy in 2012. There were no published literature reviews, no publicly distributed assessments of the evidence, no public consultations.

The IOC Medical and Scientific Commission took the same secretive approach following the CAS decision. In November 2015, it convened a secret, by-invitation-only meeting in Lausanne to consider the judgement, with six of the nine witnesses who testified before CAS in support of the Hyperandrogenism Regulations in attendance and none of the witnesses on Chand's side, and issued the aforementioned 'Consensus' statement that reiterated its support of the Regulations. While the IOC had assigned the Medical and Scientific Commission responsibility for these matters, the way in which it carried out this responsibility does not inspire confidence. Its secretive approach in the face of known differences of opinion and the presentation of a narrow range of views, developed in secret, as an international 'consensus' suggests conspiracy, not responsible public policy. It is shocking that the IOC allowed such documents to be released in its name, yet it has a long history of allowing the medical and scientific commission to issue 'consensus' statements that express a very narrow selection of views. Moreover, participation in these deliberations has always been limited to biophysical scientists. Whether the issue is 'sexual or gender identification' or 'fairness', there are outstanding scholars, scientists and ethicists from many other disciplines who could and should contribute to policy on such complex and universal subjects. Yet neither the IAAF nor the IOC have sought to broaden its examination of these issues, let alone establish a merit-based process by which members of the policy-making bodies have been chosen or check conflicts of interest. On the contrary, membership has always been drawn from a narrow circle of decision-makers with limited renewal. One of the driving forces behind the hyperandrogenism policy, Arne Ljundqvist of Sweden, a former Olympic high jumper, shaped major policy decisions for more than 40 years. He led the Swedish athletic federation from 1973 to 1981 and the Swedish Sports Confederation from 1989 to 2001 and served on the IOC from 1994 until his retirement in 2011. He chaired the IAAF medical and anti-doping commission from 1980 to 2004 and served on the IOC medical and scientific commission from 1987 to 2014, chairing that body from 2003 to 2014. While at times critical of specific tests – he came to oppose the buccal smear – throughout his long tenure he exercised an unswerving commitment to the idea of the medical regulation of female athletes. Another key player has been the French physician and exercise physiologist Stéphane Bermon. He sits on the IAAF and IOC bodies which developed the hyperandrogenism regulations, even though he conducts research into the very area in which the regulations were made, accepts funding for that research from the IAAF and was a co-author on the Fénichel paper documenting the four cases where healthy women were persuaded to undergo irreversible surgery in order to continue their athletic careers under the regulations. In other words, he is deeply invested in the policy. The IAAF's appeal is based upon a paper first authored by Bermon, commissioned by the IAAF, yet it makes no effort to seek independent advice nor separate policy-making from its sponsored research.

Inadequate evidence

The most damning finding of the CAS decision was that the IAAF had little or no evidence for the policy it imposed upon every athletic woman in the world. This was the tragic consequence of its secretive rush to judgement. Testimony before the Court established that there are few published studies examining the relationship between endogenous testosterone and performance among athletic women, the relationship that underlies the entire Regulations and even fewer when the Hyperandrogenism Regulations were promulgated in 2011 and 2012. Had the IAAF published literature reviews with the announcement of the policies, it would have had to report, as Katrina Karkazis and her colleagues did in 2012, that

Despite the many assumptions about the relationship between testosterone and athletic advantage, there is no evidence showing that successful athletes have higher testosterone levels than less successful athletes. (Karkazis, Jordan-Young, Davis and Camporesi, italics in original.)

In 2014, *three years after the IAAF policy was approved*, in a paper funded by the IAAF, Stéphane Bermon's team concluded from a study of 849 female elite athletes that:

> The lack of definitive research linking female hyperandrogenism and sporting performance is problematic and represents another central point of the controversy (9, 31). With the exception of data extracted from doping programs in female athletes in the former German Democratic Republic (7), there is no clear scientific evidence proving that a high level of T is a significant determinant of performance in female sports. (Bermon et al. 2014)

'My mind's made up–don't confuse me with the facts' has been a long-standing pattern of the medical commissions. At CAS, the veteran decision-maker Lundquist 'acknowledged that there had been a history of ignorance with respect to' previous tests (CAS 228, 65–66). Richard Holt, a witness recruited by Chand, compared the introduction of hyperandrogenism testing to that for human growth hormone. He pointed out that while tests for growth hormone were developed in the early 1990s, they were not implemented until 2012, to enable 'scientists … to establish the scientific proof needed to justify the implementation of a growth hormone testing regime'. He then went on to say that

> the present state of the scientific knowledge about the role endogenous testosterone on athletic performance is … similar to the state of knowledge about growth hormone in the 1990s (and) that the current state of the knowledge is rudimentary and there is a long way to go before the evidence can withstand scientific scrutiny. (CAS, 157, 46)

One might have hoped that with such a history, in the context of such scientific disagreement, caution was doubly required, but no – the decision-makers were determined to proceed.

Is fairness purely a matter of biology and hormones?

As the testimony to CAS reveals, IAAF policy-makers were preoccupied by the fear that some women might be approaching the male range in some biological characteristics. Nevertheless, the IAAF claimed it had abandoned 'gender verification' and 'gender policy' and was motivated purely on grounds of the fairness of women's competition, and that high testosterone gave such women an unfair advantage. The Regulations were necessary to preserve the 'level playing field' in women's sports, it argued (CAS, 250, 74). All sports officials (and athletes and coaches) should be concerned with fairness. Given that sports at the highest level are organized into male and female sectors and yet human sexuality and gender are not expressed or lived in a clear binary but across a varied spectrum, I also agree that there must be some way of defining who is male and who is female for purposes of competition. But should the medical and scientific commissions have a monopoly on these issues? Humans are not the sum of our hormones, and an understanding of human biology and biochemistry is insufficient for a complete understanding of human sexuality and human societies. Both the definition of gender and considerations of fairness in sport require social scientific, legal and ethical considerations as well as biophysical ones. This should be especially the case in a movement that recognizes the extraordinary social, economic, political, cultural and individual diversity around the world, and endeavours to promote understanding and respect for those many differences. If the exercise is to rule out the most extreme unfairness in international sport, then decision-makers should start by addressing the huge disparities in individual and national income, the most significant factors correlated to the medal list, and perhaps return to the requirement of the ancient Olympics that all athletes live and train under the same material and nutritional conditions for a set period prior to each games. The IOC and the international federations should remove the responsibility for these issues from the medical and scientific commissions and transfer any responsibility for gender definition to the women's and athletes' commissions, and for 'fairness' to the athletes' and ethics commissions.

No consultation with those affected

Throughout the CAS hearing, IAAF officials testified that they were doing it for the athletes, suggesting that the policy had been initiated in response to a broad call by athletes. There were and are athletes who believe that hyperandrogenism gives their competitors an unfair advantage, two of whom (Olympians Paula Ratcliffe and IOC medical and scientific commission member Maria-José Martinez-Patino) testified at CAS. There are also athletes who oppose the Regulations, one of whom (Olympian Madeline Pape) testified on behalf of Chand. Athletes do know and care about such issues, and in fact, it was the opposition of the IOC Athletes' Commission that finally brought 'gender verification' testing' to an end in 1999. But there was never any a systemic athlete consultation in the case of the Hyperandrogenism Regulations, especially among athletes who might have concerns about the test. It is instructive that when WADA considered regulation about hypoxic tents and altitude chambers (to neutralize the advantage that some athletes enjoy by living and training at altitude), there was a worldwide discussion involving athletes, ethicists and sports leaders from around the world (*Sydney Morning Herald* 2006). There should be such consultation in any future policy development.

No consideration of human rights

Despite the Fundamental Principles of Olympism that

> The practice of sport is a human right. Every individual must have the possibility of practising sport, without discrimination of any kind and in the Olympic spirit, which requires mutual understanding with a spirit of friendship, solidarity and fair play. (Olympic Charter, 2016, 4, 11)

And

The enjoyment of the rights and freedoms set forth in this Olympic Charter shall be secured without discrimination of any kind, such as race, colour, sex, sexual orientation, language, religion, political or other opinion, national or social origin, property, birth or other status. (Olympic Charter, 6, 12)

There is no evidence that neither the IAAF nor the IOC medical commission took these obligations into account in their deliberations. In testimony submitted to CAS, Paul Melia, the president of the Canadian Centre for Ethics in Sports, Canada's anti-doping agency, which also has responsibility for promoting sport that is fair, safe and open to all, wrote that the Hyperandrogenism Regulations were

objectionable on moral, ethical and legal grounds .... Applying the Regulations in Canada could result in a breach of national or provincial human rights or anti-discrimination legislation. The CCES does not support the Hyperandrogenism Regulations and would refuse to participate in any testing or procedures mandated under them. (CAS, 271, 80, 81)

Insensitive implementation

Finally, the Regulations were implemented without education or the training of responsible officials to ensure the fair treatment of the athletes being tested and that their confidentiality was being protected. In Chand's case, she was not told about the nature of the test which led to her suspension – she was told that she was to undergo a 'routine doping test', she was not told about the availability of appeal, and the results were leaked to the media. As she explained to CAS,

the media began reporting that Ms Chand was not permitted to compete and publicly questioned her gender. Ms Chand described her shock and devastation upon being informed that she could no longer compete. She described the severe distress she experienced as a result of the ensuing media speculation about her gender, which humiliated and 'shamed' her and her family. Ms Chand said that she felt abandoned, insecure and helpless. She was subjected to cruel questions from reporters and felt like a student who had failed her exams. Even in her rural village, she and her parents could not escape the intense and invasive media attention. (CAS, 374, 107)

A higher standard

In other spheres of regulation – in health and pharmaceuticals, the environment, education, employment, investment and so on – policy-makers are expected to establish clear standards of evidence for the rules they seek to introduce and consult with those affected before any new requirement is implemented. In the United States, for example, federal government agencies are mandated to keep the public informed about their organization, procedures and rules; provide for public participation in the rulemaking process; establish uniform standards for the conduct of formal rulemaking and adjudication; and provide for judicial review. They have been required to do so since the passage of the Administrative Procedure Act of 1946 (United States 2017). Similar safeguards are in place in many other countries, and extend to public and publicly financed programmes in sport. In Canada, the Sport Dispute Resolution Centre of Canada, which adjudicates appeals involving the national sports organizations, including the Canadian Olympic Committee, provides policy-making guidelines that stress comprehensive, well-researched rules and extensive consultation with those affected before approval and implementation (Sport Dispute Resolution Centre of Canada n.d.) The World Anti-Doping Agency conducts an annual consultation on proposed changes to the List of Prohibited Substances and Methods 'before preparing and publishing the List by 1 October in order to allow for its introduction at the start of the following year (World Anti-Doping Agency n.d.)'

I recommend that the IOC (and its member federations) follow the well-established policy making guidelines of the United Nations system, with which it enjoys Permanent Observer Status and increasingly partners in sport for development. In April 2014, the UN and the IOC signed an agreement aimed at strengthening collaboration between the two organizations, stressing that the IOC and the UN 'share the same values of contributing to a better and peaceful world through sport'. To this end, I urge the IOC to adopt the World Health Organization's *Handbook for Guideline Development* for all future policies affecting the eligibility, health and well-being of athletes. The WHO guidelines provide detailed directions for the entire chain of policy-making, from initial problem analysis through recommendation, approval, implementation, monitoring and evaluation. Among other steps, they stipulate

- Exhaustive literature reviews and syntheses
- A division of labour between an overall steering committee, a guideline development group and an external review group. The external review group should be

geographically and gender-balanced, include stakeholders and content experts … and may include groups likely to oppose or criticize the output on the basis of scientific or philosophical differences. While it may not be possible to reach agreement with them, it is important to consider their input. In addition, many of these groups and experts will play a key role in the implementation of the recommendations in the guideline; they are more likely to help implement the recommendations if they are involved from the beginning.

- Declaration and management of conflict of interests
- Careful evidence assessment, following the GRADE (Grading of Recommendations, Assessment, Development and Evaluation) approach (GRADE Working Group n.d.)
- Recommendations that weigh the quality of the evidence, the balance of benefits against harms and burdens, values and preferences and the costs of intervening (World Health Organization n.d., 9, 10)

Introducing such requirements into the procedures of the medical commissions is long overdue. While reforming the medical commissions is just one step in the ongoing task of reforming Olympic governance, it is urgently needed if the IOC is to end the long and damaging history of gender policing and the embarrassment it brings upon the Olympic Movement. I am convinced that if such procedures were in place, the Hyperandrogenism Regulations would never have been introduced.

Towards responsible autonomy in Olympic sport

My premise for this paper has been that regulators of sport, arguably the most accessible and visible form of public culture, enabled through public subsidy in every country in the world, should comply with the highest standards of transparency and accountability established for governments and other agencies with extensive public responsibilities. Some might counter that the Olympic Movement proudly asserts the 'autonomy of sport' and needs only to be responsible to itself. For example, the *Olympic Charter* declares that 'the organisation, administration and management of sport must be controlled by independent sports organisations' (Fundamental Principle 4, 11). Yet such absolute assertions of autonomy fly in the face of the realities of modern sports in the twenty-first century and only serve to distort relations with governments and the broad public. It is a given of contemporary social science that sport is constituted by intricate social processes, including the prevailing political economy; it was neither developed nor is conducted and celebrated in isolation from other social structures and practices. While most governments played only cameo roles in the Olympic sports up until the 1960s, they have been deeply, indispensably involved in the decades since, providing facilities and other infrastructure, the education and training of athletes, funds for high performance research and competition and the affirmation of public acclaim. The Olympic sports touch on many other aspects of public policy, from education and health to urban design and economic growth, as is frequently recognized. In these circumstances, governments have every right to expect that sports organizations will abide by legislation and regulations that are democratically determined (and participate in the determining processes), not just simply claim autonomy. This is not to say that sports bodies should not make their own decisions, but to do so in a way that addresses the legitimate concern about transparency and accountability.

I regard the Olympic Movement like the universities which have long prized their autonomy under the banner of academic freedom. Given the extent of public support for higher education in most countries, the universities face similar challenges and pressures. At my university, we continue to prize and work to strengthen our processes of self-government, but in a way that clearly acknowledges the constitutive power of the provincial legislature and respects and seeks to influence its oversight. We call that approach 'transparent and responsible autonomy'. It is instructive that the courts and other tribunals hearing complaints about the university will first examine 'university law' to determine whether decisions have been reasonable, just as in adjudicating complaints about sport they will first consider the decisions made under sports law. But ultimately, sports bodies as well as universities have to be accountable to public law.

It is time that the Olympic leadership take on the task of creating 'transparent and responsible autonomy' in the work of the medical and other commissions. That would be a fitting legacy of the remarkable courage of Dutee Chand.

Disclosure statement

No potential conflict of interest was reported by the author.

References

Bavington, L. D. 2016. "Regulating Hyperandrogenism in Elite Female Athletes: The History and Current Politics of Sex-control in Women's Sport." PhD thesis, University of Otago.

Beckett, A. H. 1976. "The Work of the IOC Medical Commission." In *The Olympic Games*, edited by L. Killanin and J. Rodda, 166–170. New York: Macmillan.

Bermon, S. 2017. "Androgens and Athletic Performance of Elite Female Athletes." *Current Opinion in Endocrinology, Diabetes and Obesity* 24 (3): 246–251. doi:10.1097/MED.0000000000000335.

Bermon, S., and P.-Y. Garnier. 2017. "Serum Androgen Levels and Their Relation to Performance in Track and Field: Mass Spectrometry Results from 2127 Observations in Male and Female Elite Athletes." *British Journal of Sports Medicine* 51 (17): 1309–1314. doi:10.1136/bjsports-2017-097792.

Bermon, S., P. Y. Garnier, A. L. Hirschberg, N. Robinson, S. Giraud, R. Nicoli, N. Baume, et al. 2014. "Serum Androgen Levels in Elite Female Athletes." *Journal of Clinical Endocrinology and Metabolism* 99 (11): 4328–4335. doi:10.1210/jc.2014-1391.

Canada. 1991. *International Relations Background Briefing Gender Verification*. Ottawa: Ministry of Fitness and Amateur Sport.

CAS (Court of Arbitration for Sport). 2015. *CAS 2014/a/3759 Dutee Chand v Athletics Federation of India (AFI) & International Association of Athletics Federations (IAAF). Interim Arbitral Award.* Accessed January 5, 2017. http://www.tas-cas.org/fileadmin/user_upload/award_internet.pdf

Chappelet, J.-L., and B. Kubler-Mabbott. 2008. *The International Olympic Committee and the Olympic System*. London: Routledge.

Cole, C. L. 2000. "Testing for Sex or Drugs?" *Journal of Sport and Social Issues* 24 (4): 331–333. doi:10.1177/0193723500244001.

Donnelly, P., and M. K. Donnelly. 2013. *The London 2012 Olympics: A Gender Equality Audit*. Toronto: Centre for Sport Policy Studies, University of Toronto.

Fénichal, P., F. Paris, P. Philibert, S. Hieronimus, L. Gaspari, J.-Y. Kurzenne, P. Chevallier, S. Bermon, N. Chevalier, C. Sultan, et al. 2013. "Molecular Diagnosis of 5 – Reductase Deficiency in 4 Elite Young Female Athletes through Hormonal Screening for Hyperandrogenism." *The Journal of Clinical Endocrinology & Metabolism* 98 (6): E1055–E1059. doi:10.1210/jc.2012-3893.

Ferguson-Smith, M. A., and E. Ferris. 1991. "Gender Verification in Sport: The Need for Change?" *British Journal of Sports Medicine* 25 (1): 17–20. doi:10.1136/bjsm.25.1.17.

GRADE Working Group. n.d. Accessed November 3, 2017. www.gradeworkinggroup.org

Gillespie, K. 2016a. "IOC's Gender Stance Insensitive and Harmful to Athletes." *Toronto Star*, February 23. Accessed January 7, 2017. https://www.thestar.com/sports/amateur/2016/02/23/iocs-stand-on-masculine-women-insensitive-and-harmful.html

Gillespie, K. 2016b. "No New Rules Planned: IOC Confirms It Won't Act on Hyperandrogenism Issue, but Indian Sprinter Remains Wary." *Toronto Star*, February 26. Accessed January 7, 2017. http://www.pressreader.com/canada/toronto-star/20160226/282587377053651

Henne, K. 2014. "The 'Science' of Fair Play in Sport: Gender and the Politics of Testing." *Signs* 39 (3): 787–812. doi:10.1086/674208.

IAAF (International Association of Athletics Federations). n.d. "IAAF Historical Milestones." Accessed January 15, 2017. https://www.iaaf.org/about-iaaf/history

IOC. 2015. *Olympic Solidarity 2015 Annual Report*. Accessed January 15, 2017. https://stillmed.olympic.org/media/Document%20Library/OlympicOrg/IOC/Who-We-Are/Commissions/Olympic-Solidarity/2015-Report-A-Direct-Line.pdf#_ga=1.109754508.821534916.1473127867

IOC. n.d. "Nine Centres Worldwide Now Recognized as IOC Research Centres for the Prevention of Injury and the Protection of Athletes' Health." Accessed January 15, 2017. https://www.olympic.org/news/nine-centres-worldwide-recognised-as-ioc-research-centres-for-prevention-of-injury-and-protection-of-athlete-health

IOC (International Olympic Committee). 2016. *IOC Consensus Meeting on Sex Reassignment and Hyperandrogenism November 2015*. Medical and Scientific Commission. Accessed January 7, 2017. https://stillmed.olympic.org/media/Document%20Library/OlympicOrg/IOC/Who-We-Are/Commissions/Medical-and-Scientific-Commission/EN-IOC-Consensus-Meeting-on-Sex-Reassignment-and-Hyperandrogenism.pdf#_ga=2.83943961.1069172592.1494257701-1631448284.1447421530

Karkazis, K., and R. Jordan-Young. 2013. "The Harrison Bergeron Olympics." *American Journal of Bioethics* 13 (t5): 66–69. doi:10.1080/15265161.2013.776375.

Karkazis, K., and G. Meyerowitz-Katz. 2017. "Why the IAAF's Latest Testosterone Study Won't Help Them at CAS." *World Sports Advocate*. Accessed August 28, 2017. http://www.cecileparkmedia.com/world-sports-advocate/hottopic.asp?id=1525

Karkazis, K., R. Jordan-Young, G. Davis, and S. Camporesi. 2012. "Out of Bounds? A Critique of the New Policies on Hyperandrogenism in Elite Female Athletes." *American Journal of Bioethics* 12 (7): 2–16. doi:10.1080/15265161.2012.680533.

Kolata, G. 2010. "IOC Panel Calls for Treatment in Sex Ambiguity Cases." *The New York Times*, January 20. Accessed January 29, 2017. http://www.nytimes.com/2010/01/21/sports/olympics/21ioc.html

Lenskyj, H. J. 2013. *Gender Politics and the Olympic Industry*. New York: Palgrave MacMillan.

Mitra, P. 2015. "Governance Challenges at the National Level." *Play the Game, Aarhus, Denmark*, October 28.

New, M., and J. L. Simpson, eds. 2011. *Hormonal and Genetic Basis of Sexual Differentiation Disorders and Hot Topics in Endocrinology: Proceedings of the 2nd World Conference*. New York: Springer.

Nolen, S. 2016. "How India's Dutee Chand Ran past Gender Barriers to Compete in Rio." *Globe and Mail*, August 12. Accessed January 7, 2017. https://beta.theglobeandmail.com/sports/olympics/how-indias-dutee-chand-ran-past-gender-barriers-to-compete-in-rio/article31385923/?ref=http://www.theglobeandmail.com

Padawer, R. 2016. "The Humiliating Practice of Sex Testing Female Athletes." *New York times Magazine*, June 28. Accessed January 7, 2017. https://www.nytimes.com/2016/07/03/magazine/the-humiliating-practice-of-sex-testing-female-athletes.html?mcubz=3

Patino, M.-J. M. 2005. "Personal Account: A Woman Tried and Tested." *The Lancet* 366: S38, December.

Pieper, L. P. 2014. "Sex Testing and the Maintenance of Western Femininity in International Sport." *International Journal of the History of Sport* 31 (13): 1557–1576.

Press Trust of India. 2017. "Dutee Chand's Case to Be Reopened." *The Hindu*, July 4. Accessed July 6, 2017. http://www.thehindu.com/sport/athletics/dutee-chands-gender-case-to-be-re-opened/article19209339.ece#!

Ritchie, I. 2003. "Sex Tested, Gender Verified: Controlling Female Sexuality in the Age of Containment." *Sport History Review* 34: 80–98.

Schultz, J. 2011. "Caster Semenya and the 'Question of Too': Sex Testing in Elite Women's Sport and the Issue of Advantage." *Quest* 63: 228–243. doi:10.1080/00336297.2011.10483678.

Slater, M. 2015. "A History of Bad Science and 'Biological Racism'." *BBC Sports*, July 28. Accessed January 7, 2017. http://www.bbc.com/sport/athletics/29446276

Sonksen, P., M. A. Ferguson-Smith, L. D. Bavington, R. I. G. Holt, D. A. Cowan, D. H. Catlin, B. Kidd, et al. 2015. "Medical and Ethical Concerns regarding Women with Hyperandrogenism and Elite Sport." *Journal of Clinical Endocrinology and Metabolism* 100: 825–827, Early Release, January 14. doi:10.1210/jc.2014-3206.

Sport Dispute Resolution Centre of Canada. n.d. *Selection Criteria for Major Events in Sports: Guidelines and Tips*. Accessed May 7, 2017. http://www.crdsc-sdrcc.ca/eng/documents/SDRCC_PolicyDoc_Selection_ENG_web.pdf

United Nations. 2016. Human Rights Council, *Report of the Special Rapporteur on the right of Everyone to the Enjoyment of the Highest Attainable Standard of Physical and Mental Health, a/HRC/32/33, April 4*, 16.

United States. 2017. *The Administrative Procedure Act, 1946*. Accessed May 7, 2017. https://www.epa.gov/laws-regulations/summary-administrative-procedure-act

Wells, C. 2010. "Diagnosing Sex-gender Verification and the IOC." In *Proceedings of the 10th International Symposium on Olympic Research*, 301–311. London: Olympic Studies Centre, University of Western Ontario.

World Anti-Doping Agency. n.d. "Prohibited List." Accessed May 7, 2017. https://www.wada-ama.org/en/what-we-do/prohibited-list

World Health Organization. n.d. *WHO Handbook on Guideline Development*. Geneva: WHO Press. Accessed May 7, 2017. http://apps.who.int/iris/bitstream/10665/75146/1/9789241548441_eng.pdf

Canada 2015: perceptions and experiences of the organisation and governance of the Women's World Cup

Carrie Dunn

ABSTRACT

Just as female fans have been ignored, there has also been a tradition of women's football in England being equally invisibilized, most obviously in studies and media which purport to present a full history of the game. That includes the way it is treated by the game's governors. FIFA has a strange ambivalence to its leading female football practitioners. Much of the run-up to the 2015 Women's World Cup was overshadowed by the decision to play the tournament on artificial pitches rather than grass, and the threats of legal action from a group of high-profile players. However, the tournament was also the biggest ever, with an expanded number of teams, and an additional round-of-16 before the quarter-finals. This paper discusses fans' perceptions and direct experiences of the 2015 Women's World Cup, whether in person or by following the tournaments via the media coverage. Based on my original qualitative interview data gathered in Canada during the tournament, it is increasingly clear that there was a significant amount of fan dissatisfaction around the planning and scheduling of the matches and the organisation and publicity of the tournament as a whole, much of it directed at FIFA. Several people suggested that the Women's World Cup is treated as less important and interesting by the governing body, by the media and the public at large simply because it is a women's tournament and thus perceived as second-rate.

Introduction

Women's football in England has been invisibilized and sidelined away from the 'mal-estream' (Dunn, 2014, 2); it is treated as lesser, as abnormal and as unworthy of attention. That includes the way it is treated by the game's governing bodies, often with a bewildering nonchalance or ambivalence to its most high-profile practitioners. The months leading up to the 2015 Women's World Cup in Canada were dominated not by match previews and squad selections, but by the threat of legal action from players who objected to FIFA's insistence that they should play the tournament on artificial pitches rather than grass, arguing that senior male players would never have to do that. Despite that, this international tournament was expanding globally, with more teams taking part, necessitating an additional round-of-16 before the quarter-finals.

Next to no research currently exists on fans of women's football. Even though individual experiences are now being reported and listened to, the football fan is still assumed to be male; and football is still assumed to be a 'man's game', with institutional sexism still pervasive. The apparent anxiety to attract women, children and family groups to men's football is not due to a keenness to promote equality of opportunity, but to maximize ticket revenues and merchandise spend. The same applies to football more broadly, as attendees or as participants. Indeed, research over the past three decades has begun to report on the diversity of football crowds (mostly looking at men's football), but also the different forms of sexism still present in the stadium and in the structures of the game as a whole, broadly preventing women's participation as players, fans and administrators (see Dunn 2014, for further detail). The exploration of the experience of (both male and female) fans of women's football is thus a new tangent for the field.

This paper draws on my research before and during the 2015 Women's World Cup; respondents completed a questionnaire prior to the tournament, and a smaller group were selected for qualitative interview, mostly in person in Canada, although some were via Skype if they were watching matches in a different host city. (See Dunn 2015, for a full account of this research project.)

The tradition of invisibility

In England, the ban on women playing football on FA-affiliated pitches came into play in 1921, and stood for half a century. Even after it was lifted, the FA were still hesitant to take on the governance of the women's game, leaving that to the Women's FA, who they invited to affiliate with them, just as a county FA would do. During their tenure, a representative England team participated in some international tournaments, but with the rules modified – for example, two halves of 40 min were played in the Mundialito, contested during the 1980s. UEFA and FIFA have endorsed international women's football competition only relatively recently. Independently operated international tournaments were attracting crowds of over 10,000 in the 1960s and 1970s, and UEFA was evidently concerned about the possibility of losing control of a popular form of football competition, despite their efforts to stay as far removed from it as possible in the preceding decades. FIFA members were instructed in 1970 that they should take control of the women's game amidst fears that external organisations and people were profiting financially from it (see Williams 2013 for more detail).

Yet the resultant actions were not immediate. In 1971, UEFA's member organizations voted 39–1 in favour of national associations taking control of the women's game, with Scotland the sole association voting against (Lopez 1997, 59). It took until 1975 to establish the Asian Cup, with an Oceania equivalent following in 1983. World tournaments were finally established in the late 1980s following a series of 'world invitationals'; China hosted an unofficial women's World Cup in 1988 as well as the first official tournament in 1991 (Lopez 1997, 195); and in 1996 women's football was adopted as an Olympic sport (Williams 2013, 12).

Fans' experience of the governance of the 2015 Women's World Cup

It is perhaps not surprising, given this history, that Women's World Cups still struggle to make an impact on the sports media consciousness. Annie, an England fan based in the USA, thought that people had a general lack of awareness that the tournament was happening, even in Canada itself, partially because of the choice of the host cities. She said that the small east coast town Moncton was an unusual and problematic choice as a venue, explaining:

> When I got to the airport and went through immigration, the immigration officer said why are you in Canada, and I was like, 'I'm here to watch the World Cup,' and he was like, 'Oh, yeah, I heard that was going on, maybe I'll try to catch a game.' That doesn't happen in the men's World Cup. People just don't know. I guess if they were trying to span those stadiums across the country, Moncton's kind of a weird location for it, given the size of the stadium and that it's on a college campus...the tickets weren't sold out for today, they were saying there's a few hundred left...Would it have been sold out if it was in Toronto or Winnipeg? People want to see England and France.

However, Moncton was not the only host city that found itself with problems; fans who watched games in the bigger cities also reported a lack of publicity around the tournament as well as a less-than-ideal approach to matchday organization. USA fan Cassie also felt some of the media coverage of the tournament was patronizing, and criticized the anthropomorphized mascot for the tournament, an owl clearly marked as female with very long eyelashes and pink 'lipstick' around her beak. She said:

> When I was in Winnipeg the city seemed small. It just didn't seem like it was equipped to handle or even believed that it was handling a world-class event. There was a sense of there's this throwaway event that's happening over in Winnipeg Stadium, so you get there and it's all American fans, which is great, and obviously we know how to mobilize, but yeah, it felt small, and then over to Vancouver, which is supposed to be the crowning jewel of the tournament, and it still felt small at BC Place. 55,000 fans, that's great, but it didn't feel - on some level it feels patronising in terms of the way that even the sport is spoken about and the way the sport has been treated up in Canada, like oh, look at this cute little event, and look at this furry owl with lipstick mascot that we have, and look at how great those girls are doing, that sort of thing. That's just sort of the general vibe I'm getting from it, and it just feels like a step backwards from what I experienced in '99... all of these decisions that have been made, whether it comes to what we talked about before with the draw, to six time zones, why the hell is it spread across six time zones, that makes no sense, all of these decisions that are being made for quote unquote marketing and promotional reasons as opposed to foster competition, that's the most insulting thing you could possibly do to a world-class event, because you basically walk into it and you concede that no-one cares about this, and so we have to make all of these decisions, who cares about equal playing field and maximizing the level of competition by making things fair for everyone? Let's make all of these concessions because we already come in defeated as FIFA, we don't think anybody's going to be watching this.

Cassie is implying that the Women's World Cup is simply not seen as important or as elite international sporting competition. She mentions that the seeding and fixtures were adjusted to maximize viewing audiences as far as possible rather than relying on the luck of the draw as is usual in tournaments; and she suggests that FIFA were not expecting anyone to be interested in the tournament simply for its own sake. The effort to put France and England in the same group with matches on the east coast (and thus just a five-hour time difference with London, six with Paris) was a point raised by several respondents; and even those who understood or accepted the reasoning about expanding the international television coverage felt that playing the games in Moncton, at a university sports field with temporary stands, showed a lack of consideration or planning. Danielle, a Canadian fan who lived on the east coast of the country, said:

> When it comes to sports games, it's been a bone of contention because Halifax is a way bigger city and a huge, much larger market [than Moncton], but we don't have a proper stadium. So having the game at Moncton was pitch-wise the equivalent of doing it at a major university, you just happen to have more seats, because they have redone that stadium to host games from the under-20s [U20s Women's World Cup] last year, so when it comes to getting events, Moncton definitely is more clever, but I thought that geographically it's so far removed. Like, the games for the World Cup, Canada is way too big of a country to host something like that when fans have absolutely no possibility of going to all the games or even a variety. Canada played their first two games in Alberta. Alberta is an eight-hour flight [from the east coast of Canada], and it would cost three thousand, four thousand dollars to get there, and then Montreal [for the third and final group game], people from here, I do know people who are going to the Montreal game on Monday, so the whole idea and I guess in practice of getting games to the East Coast was great because we do have quite a big soccer market here, but just the actual application of it was just garbage.

Danielle's knowledge of the towns and cities on the Canadian east coast gives her anecdote a certain increased weighting, as she emphasizes that Moncton is a venue unsuitable for hosting a major tournament; and suggests that more fans would have been attracted had the games been scheduled in a bigger, i.e. more easily accessible, town or city on the east coast. She also highlights how difficult it would be for fans to follow a team throughout the tournament (i.e. from group stage to final) because of the sheer distance between the host cities, and the expense it would accrue (and she notes that Canadians would find it equally difficult to follow their national team rather than having a home advantage). Danielle also has additional authority as she had actually attended a game in Moncton, and had criticisms of the match day organization, explaining:

> We got to where they held the game at, Universite de Moncton, it was at the local university, and they had sold parking passes, but there was only like a hundred, they were charging 20 dollars, they sold out really quickly and then they said, 'Well, no problem, everyone park at the Moncton Coliseum' - which is a local sports arena – 'and there will be shuttles that will take you to the university,' so when we got there, which was, well, kick-off was 2, we got there around 20 to 1, there was probably maybe five, six hundred people in front of us, and there were three, like, regular school-bus size buses going back and forth, and the drive there and back was 20 min. So imagine, gosh, maximum, there was one, like, proper coach, so the max that would hold would be like 50 people, so within a 20-min span they were only moving 40 people there and back, so by the time we got there to the university it was 25 past 2, we missed the first goal, we missed almost the entire first half, and I would say that behind us in the queue to get shuttles there was probably 4,000 people, who would have completely missed the first game, and probably a lot of them even parts of the second game. There would have been no way they would have gotten everyone there on time. It was ridiculous, and I thought organisation-wise it was a no-brainer. You know how many tickets you sell, you know how many parking passes were sold, so do the math and you have 11,000 people who need to get to the university, so three buses on a 20-min return journey is not going to get 11,000 people there, and there was no other transportation - people were calling cabs from the queue to get on the shuttles.

Mark, an England fan living in Canada, agreed with Danielle's criticism of the event planning in Moncton for the first group games. After the situation Danielle had described, officials were quoted in the media referring to people arriving at the ground only in time for kick-off, due to 'a little bit of a maritime laid-back approach', suggesting that all the fans who were there were locals. Mark had been in these queues, but disagreed with the official line; he said that the problems were not with the fans but with the lackadaisical approach of the event organisers. He said:

> At the moment there are quite a lot of problems going around, financial kind of problems in the province, and there's a lack of business and opportunity here, and I think that's the kind of attitude that fosters that kind of approach, oh, we're all laidback and chilled out here, we're just small-time people, the FIFA World Cup is a, it's a really big event and we're really lucky to have it but you know, we're chilled and laidback and not going to take it seriously. That's kind of very patronizing, I feel, because there are a lot of very serious people here, and there's a lot of very business-oriented people, and it's kind of frustrating to see that that attitude still remains. I think the people there were, I guess, kind of taken by surprise. It is kind of a little bit, a lot of what we've been talking about in the build-up to the World Cup has been about the difference between the women's World Cup and the men's World Cup. The men would never have to play on 3G pitches, and similarly within the men's game it would be unacceptable to have people who have lined up for an hour and be 30 min late. That, I find, kind of, yeah, I mean, if this was the men's World Cup that would be totally unacceptable and that would be a huge story, a very very big deal, and for them to come out and say oh, we're kind of laidback, I think that's definitely not good enough.

The implication here is that the problems with organization were covered up without too much criticism in the media because the game the fans were waiting to see was one contested by women.

Fans' experience of ticketing at the 2015 Women's World Cup

Annie talked about her travels to watch England's group games, which did not require a significant amount of preparation; indeed, she had only been planning her trip for the previous two weeks. She clarified: 'In my head, [I have been planning it for] a really long time. My wife is American and one of my best friends is Canadian, so we talked about it four years ago, after the last World Cup – 'Wherever the next one is, we'll go.' When tickets went on sale, I'd just started a job and didn't have a lot of time off and thought I really couldn't make it happen, and so I just said to myself, 'Oh, we'll just watch it on TV, we'll have friends over,' and then about a month ago I was in England and started to see all the hype, and thought, 'I've got to go, I've got to go.' My wife couldn't come so I was like I'll find someone else who wants to go, so I asked [my friend Bonnie], and two weeks ago we booked our tickets, so really it was the last four years, since Germany ended, but really only two weeks ago.'

If Annie was able to buy tickets for the Women's World Cup just a week or two before the matches, that would imply a lack of interest (i.e. the matches were not sold out); but on a more positive note it also reflects the reasonable pricing, as she did not have to save up to purchase them as she might have done for a men's tournament. The tickets for elite international women's football are not accorded the same high prices as the men's equivalent, as they are not seen as high demand; one wonders, perhaps, if the low-key nature of the publicity and organisation described by respondents reinforces this low demand for tickets. The concurrent events around the tournament – the tourist provision, the fan-zones, the decoration in the host cities – were also reported by respondents to be much more low profile than would be expected in the men's World Cup, creating a less exciting (perhaps less carnival) atmosphere.

Lisa described her experience of the host cities in the first fortnight of the tournament, saying: 'It feels a lot more low-key so far, it is early days, there are banners, and some pubs and restaurants have got signs out front that show that they're World Cup-friendly if you want to watch a match in their pub, but it seems a lot more low-key to me, and it's kind of disappointing. The first match that opened the stadium, the BC Place Stadium, didn't have any sort of a ceremony; we always arrive as early as we can for a match, and there were no vendors outside the stadium, and the inside of the stadium was apparently stripped down to represent only things that align with FIFA. I've never been to BC Place but that's what one of the BC Place employees commented to my friend Anne, that they really stripped it down, so getting there early meant we sat there in an empty stadium in an empty field. Usually we watch players warm up, and we did get to see some of that, but there was no recognition of opening the stadium, so it was sort of pointless to go early to an opening World Cup match, I've never had that experience before'.

Lisa suggests that the lack of glamour and publicity around the Women's World Cup reflects the way women's football has been neglected by the governing bodies, who choose instead to focus their efforts elsewhere. It is clear that during the summer of 2015 there was a significant amount of fan dissatisfaction around the planning and scheduling of the matches – and these were the people who had made the effort to travel to Canada to follow the tournament. Much of their disgruntlement was directed at FIFA, with several people suggesting that the Women's World Cup was treated as less important and interesting simply because it is a women's tournament.

Media coverage of the 2015 Women's World Cup

Of course, this criticism is not a new one. The issues around attitudes to women's sport and the coverage of women's sporting events are not problems confined to sport; they reflect societies in which women and women's achievements are still treated and perceived as lesser, whether explicitly or implicitly. This principle is reflected in the UK media's coverage of the 2015 Women's World Cup and women's football more broadly.

Someone writing about women's football as a labour of love can perhaps be forgiven for choosing to follow the games on television rather than heading to Canada in person. However, this was the attitude of many UK media outlets as well. Print outlets were loath to send staff journalists to another continent to cover the tournament, relying on freelancers and agency reports where possible. In terms of broadcast, the BBC and British Eurosport both showed matches throughout the tournaments. However, as with many sporting events, the numbers of on-site staff were relatively limited; although high-profile presenter Jacqui Oatley fronted the BBC's coverage, with studio pundits including former England inter-nationals Rachel Brown-Finnis and Rachel Yankey, they were still in the UK. The BBC's commentary team Jonathan Pearce and Sue Smith covered the England matches in Canada; but other commentary duos were based in the UK and commentating by following a live feed of the games. This kind of coverage can ever only offer a limited perspective; obviously firstly on the games being broadcast, reliant on the host broadcaster's decisions for the images displayed, but also more broadly - if reporters are not there in person, they cannot spot news stories or ask questions, meaning they are likely to rely on press releases and statements as well as official press conferences, often led by a FIFA official, reflecting the threat of 'churnalism' identified by Davies (2009) is clear.

Many news outlets opted to use 'user-generated content' to bolster their coverage, particularly for their online provision – asking fans who were actually there to send in pictures, video and comment so that their journalists (back in the UK) could turn them into a story. Even the well-respected BBC was not immune to this. One respondent reported in interview: 'We're on Twitter, and the BBC put out a thing saying if you're going [to the Women's World Cup], download this app and you can send us your photos, and [when we downloaded the app] we started getting emails from them with their wishlist, can you go and find this person or that person? No, we're not doing that'. Her companion added: 'We embraced the BBC thing at first, sent a few shots. Because we did that, [then they asked] "Can you do this this and this?"' She added: '"Can you interview [a player's relative]?' No! For a start I wouldn't know where to start. As a fan I don't think like you think'.

These exchanges highlight some of the problems for the UK media in covering the tournament. The BBC obviously acknowledged the need and demand for multimedia content, especially human interest stories involving the England players and their families, but their limited resources meant they were not able to cover everything. Instead, they hoped that fans would be able to generate this free content to use throughout the tournament via this app.

The BBC and other outlets realized quickly that British audiences were keen for news from the Women's World Cup, but they really should not have been surprised. Over the past decade there has been a clear appetite in the UK for the broadcast of women's international tournaments involving England; for example, Bell (2012, 358) reports that the 2005 European Championship, hosted in England, was much better supported than the organizers had anticipated, and during the 2011 Women's World Cup a public outcry forced the BBC to air England's quarter-final against France on a free-to-air channel rather than online only or via the digital 'red button'. (Bell also points out in the same article that viewing figures for women's football on free-to-air channels are consistently good; when the matches are only broadcast on niche digital subscription channels, it is unsurprising that the viewing figures are vastly smaller.)

My research supported the idea that fans in the UK expected good and comprehensive coverage of the tournament from the British media. Questionnaire respondents who were not travelling to Canada made additional statements on how much they were looking forward to the TV coverage in the summer of 2015, with comments such as 'I will be watching every moment on BBC.' The England team's progress through the summer resulted in increased interest and viewing figures; and the Football Association reported at the end of the tournament that the UK viewing figures for England matches had increased by 185 per cent from the previous tournaments, with a total of 14.6 million people watching their seven games during the tournament. The third-place play-off match against Germany was watched by 2.28 million viewers, slightly down from the 2.38 million people who watched the semi-final against Japan a few days before. They also announced that the overall average audience for a match was 1.6 million - 81 per cent higher than the average of 890,000 in 2013 (across three games) and 329 per cent higher than the 380,000 (also three games) from the last World Cup in 2011 (TheFA.com, 2015b).

This boost in interest and viewing figures was reflected across the world, with fans globally noting the developments in media coverage; one questionnaire respondent highlighted with pleasure the introduction of an official tournament sticker book, just as the men's World Cup has. The official FIFA news releases confirmed this, reporting that the global viewing figures had broken records throughout the tournament; for the final, an average audience of 25.4 million fans in the United States watched their team beat Japan 5–2 live on FOX, the best viewing figures for any football match broadcast on US television, even higher than the 2014 record set during the men's World Cup when the USA played Portugal. They also reported that the Spanish-language channel Telemundo attracted a further 1.3 million viewers in the United States – the most watched Women's World Cup match on record for Spanish-language television in the United States. Even in Japan – where viewers might have been forgiven for switching off fairly promptly after the USA took such a quick lead – their broadcaster Fuji TV drew an average audience of 11.6 million for the game, compared to an audience of 9.8 million for the 2011 final, when Japan won the title. FIFA also pointed to the greater consumption of social media, reporting that the tournament's official Facebook page had a 97 per cent increase in followers, with 97.8 million impressions; Twitter followers for the official account @FIFAWWC increased by 67 per cent, generating 124.9 million impressions; and Instagram followers increased by 29 per cent, with over 1.3 million fans following the account by the end of the Women's World Cup (FIFA.com, 2015). This interest in the Women's World Cup is not a surprise even though attendances at domestic fixtures are not necessarily huge; as Hallmann's (2011: 37) work has previously observed, public opinion of the Women's World Cup is higher and more favourable than women's football generally.

Fans' feelings about women's football

During interviews with England fans, it became increasingly clear that many followed women's football as a deliberate choice, contrasting it with elements of men's football that they disliked. Joe described why he likes women's football thus: 'There's less aggression, there's less lumping long balls forward, there's more emphasis on skill and flair play, and it's a cliché but it's true, you just don't see the prima donna antics instances of the men's Premiership in the women's game. It doesn't happen. These are real people playing for the love of the game, even the few full-time pros making a realistic wage, so your fan can relate more to the female player, definitely'.

Lina also felt strongly about the importance of players' conduct, explaining that she had stopped watching men's football because of the players' off-field behaviour: 'I do like football, but I have to be honest I've become more and more frustrated with it over the last few years with the actions of players, the overall, I find it much harder to support the England men's team because there's so many of the players that I find frankly objectionable'.

Rose did not speak explicitly about players' behaviour but about the styles of play, explaining that what attracted her to women's football was '[j]ust the style of the game, with the women's game a bit slower, it might be perceived to not be as aggressive, not the same sort of fast pace, really. I think you've just got to get your head round that and you'll see that they're just as skilful, it's just as enjoyable to watch, if you separate the two types of game. It's a bit like men's and women's tennis. You watch men's tennis and it's pretty much just forearm smash smash smash, very fast-paced; you watch the women's game and you get a lot more rallies, slower pace, so that's how I see it, really'.

Almost 20 years previously, former footballer Sue Lopez (1997, 208) had reported exactly the same feelings from male fans of women's football, who preferred the slower pace of the game because it reminded them of men's football before it became 'so professional and commercialised'. One can almost perceive a philosophical division between the two 'types' of the game – but where the negative qualities are all associated with the men's game, when usually it is women's sport associated with negativity. Additionally, this contrasts with the ways in which the women's side of traditionally British sports are usually defined and described. So often players, commentators and fans are at pains to point out the *similarities* of the games, to increase the status of the women's sport, drawing equivalences with the men's. For example, Wright and Clarke's (1999, 239) analysis of the coverage of women's rugby in England shows a discourse which describes the men's and women's versions of the game as similar, and the players as similar in their behaviour – on and off the pitch, from how hard they tackle to how hard they drink.

However, this effort to idealize the game, imposing a narrative on it, also creates a problem for women's football, as it casts both women and the women's game as simply 'morally good' where men are not, rather than just treating both as sport, and their participants as human with various flaws. Football scholars have long argued for encouraging more women to attend men's games because their 'civilising' presence would encourage men to behave and thus remove the issue of hooliganism; it seems now from these responses that fans are suggesting that the women's game deserves more support because of their 'moral goodness', their honesty, their good behaviour.

Joe's description is particularly interesting; he talks about women's football and its players as the descendants of the Corinthian tradition, there purely for the love of the game, and ignoring any mercenary rewards which would sully the simplicity of their sport. It is very reminiscent of Williams's (2013, 99) conclusion that women's football relies on the perceived good qualities of its players in order to promote itself. It may not have been emphasized, but all the England players in the squad for 2015 were professional footballers (except for Claire Rafferty, who has opted to continue to work part-time as a financial analyst). The discourse of the brave, committed amateur, though, permeates the discourse around women's football in England; partly because professionalization is a relatively recent phenomenon, but it also suits those involved in the sport to create that additional distance between the men's and women's games, creating this narrative of honesty and commitment around the women to contrast them with the men almost as a marketing tactic. As respondent Rose says, it is a different style of play entirely; emphasizing the difference also emphasizes that it is not a choice between men's and women's football, and that one can enjoy both or either. Part of the attraction of women's football is the opportunity to engage directly with players, and if as Joe says part of the appeal is thinking that these elite athletes are 'real people', just like the rest of us, then that façade must be maintained through the official narratives.

In contrast to the England fans, female American and Canadian fans of women's football were established fans of women's football. As Markovits and Hellerman (2003, 14) point out, women's football tends to succeed in countries where the sport has not already been occupied by men and this is certainly the case in the North American region. Many of the younger respondents spoke about playing football as children and then progressing to watching women's football. Charlotte was a good example, saying:

> I started playing when I was five, that was definitely the first one, I was on a kiddy league
> with my twin brother, and my dad coached, and it was just a bunch of five-year-olds running
> around, and trying to kick the ball in some direction, and then you know, stuck through it,
> had a good time, got on a girls' team that my mum was the assistant coach for, and fairly soon
> I shot up, I hit 5′ 11″ in the sixth grade, when I was, you know, like, 11, and so I'd always been
> fairly tall, and also a little bit chubby, and so of course fairly quickly it was like try goal, but I
> loved it, and it totally worked, and so I played consistently from five years old till 16, and then

that was the point, in my local women's soccer, either you are committed enough to join the upper level travelling team or you're no longer playing soccer, and I was like there weren't enough people like me who were like, well, I don't have the time enough for that, but I still want to play soccer, so that was the only two years of my life where I didn't play regularly on a team, I played junior varsity in high school, I played in college, even got on a team when I studied abroad in London, and went to graduate school and immediately during orientation I overheard two women talking about soccer and I was like, soccer, are you on a team, do you need a goalkeeper? Had been playing in local women's leagues weekly for the last six or so years, so playing is a big part of it, but it was right place, right time, because I turned 13 in 1999.

Charlotte is talking here about the USA side winning the 1999 Women's World Cup, describing it as the right place (i.e. a tournament hosted in America) and the right time (i.e. when she was old enough to understand and appreciate what she was seeing). Heather, a generation older, was less influenced by the recent achievements of the USA women's team, and had begun her football career as many other women of a similar age did in Europe and in North America – playing alongside boys because there were no girls' teams to join. She recalled:

I'm 40 now, and I started playing, I was probably 5 or 6 years old. Of course we didn't have any girls' teams, so played with the boys, beat up on them a little bit, for me, I think the best thing to say about it for me is I really fell in love with the game. I found my home, so to speak, it was the place where I belonged. It was on the soccer pitch. It just grew from there. I actually took time away from the game, just moving, and life, and did different sports, and when I came to Portland, this was probably about eight, almost nine years ago, I started playing again. Portland is a fantastic city for football, and we're just very fortunate to have the kind of fanbase that we do for men's and women's football, it's a very special city, adult leagues all over the place and it's a real big community here, again, it's kind of like finding my home again.

Danielle, a Canada fan in her 30s, had grown up watching women's football, indicating that the sport had historically been taken seriously in that country (as Hall 2003, confirms) although she had not played it herself in adulthood. She said: 'I'm a huge soccer fan. I'm a Manchester City fan. My husband's from Scotland and he lived in England for years, he's actually an Arsenal and a Portsmouth fan, I'm a Portsmouth fan too, but different divisions, and I've followed soccer pretty much my whole life, I played as a kid, but I'm borderline obsessive about it. I live in the wrong country to be a football enthusiast…I've followed women's football for years. Canadians are, when it comes to sport, there's a lot of fair-weather fans because of the patriotic aspect of it, so people who might not ever watch football ever, like including the MLS, which is the closest we have to Premier League here, they won't watch, but when it comes to Olympic sports or World Cup sports, they will watch, but I've watched women's football since I was a kid, really, both Canadian and American because the American team was always just superior, and I've followed a lot of the England team in the past year especially because there's five [Manchester] City [her Premier League team] players on the England national team, so that's always interesting, but it's really a patriotic thing, if you love soccer or football, and when it comes to anything that Canada can win over the US, everyone just jumps on the bandwagon'.

Hall (2003, 30) defines football as the 'game of choice' for girls under the age of 14 in Canada, and this assertion is supported by Canadian respondents. It is significant to note here that the American and Canadian narratives focus on the competition and success in women's football as an attraction, as one might expect of any sport, but they lack the English respondents' deliberate, explicit contrasts with men's football. This is most likely because in the North America region 'soccer' has often been treated as a women's sport rather than one with all the connotations of working-class masculinity that it has in England.

Conclusion

The research showcased in this article is of course only a very tiny, self-selecting snapshot of the fans who followed the Women's World Cup in 2015; it has focused primarily on England fans, with additional interviews with those following the USA and Canada, employing that data for colour and for contrast. Nevertheless, it is a good starting point for the necessary and long neglected research into fans of women's football. Respondents from all over the world highlighted the problems the game has faced in their country, from lack of funding to lack of media coverage; but also spoken at length about the great memories and rewarding experiences they have gained from their fandom.

Few of the England fans in Canada had travelled to watch the team's matches previously, either at home or abroad, whereas the USA fans had revelled in their country hosting two previous Women's World Cups and had a firmly held tradition of following their national team. This may of course also indicate that a successful team can consistently attract more fans to a stadium than a less successful one; but it correlates to the contrast between respondents in the UK and in the North Americas on the reasons they began following women's football as outlined in this chapter. Women's football in the North Americas has a legitimacy that it simply has not had and still does not have in the UK; it is a sporting option for all children, and its profile is reasonably high. In the UK, despite increasing efforts in the past decade, it remains a niche sport, which girls of previous generations have not been encouraged to pursue, and thus they have been unaware of the women's football pyramid of leagues which, with and without FA backing, have been operating for decades. Therefore they have not known about it in order to support it – either as a participant or as a fan.

Unfortunately, negative judgement still permeates attitudes towards women's football. The FA published a survey during the 2015 Women's World Cup which indicated that fathers with young daughters held a number of negative perceptions about the sport's suitability for girls: 22 per cent expressed the view that football is a game for men, 19 per cent felt women's football was of poor quality, 17 per cent were concerned that girls would get hurt playing football, and 16 per cent even described the game as 'unladylike'. These views are not so far from that famous FA declaration in 1921, which said, 'The game of football is quite unsuitable for females and ought not to be encouraged'. Indeed, 19 per cent of fathers doubted that girls were interested in football at all (TheFA.com, 2015a). Such a declaration is surely partially a self-fulfilling prophecy; if girls are not encouraged from an early age to play or watch football, then they are less likely to do so.

Football certainly continues to have a problem with sexism, but this is because the same problems exist in the society which creates and hosts it; sexism and misogyny permeate everyday life so it is not surprising that the same prejudices are found in football. Yet, to look ahead, football could be one way in which these problems could begin to be faced, challenged and combated. The increased profile and importance of tournaments such as the Women's World Cup could prove to be significant, encouraging new generations of participants but also in establishing new generations of fans, whose attendance (and money) will maintain the game for decades to come.

Disclosure statement

No potential conflict of interest was reported by the author.

References

Bell, B. 2012. "Levelling the Playing Field? Post-Euro 2005 Development of Women's Football in the North-West of England." *Sport in Society: Cultures, Commerce, Media, Politics* 15 (3): 349–368.

Davies, N. 2009. *Flat Earth News*. London: Vintage.

Dunn, C. 2014. *Female Football Fans: Community, Identity and Sexism*. London: Palgrave Pivot.

Dunn, C. 2015. *Football and the Women's World Cup: Organisation, Media and Fandom*. London: Palgrave Pivot.

FIFA.com. 2015. "World Cup Final Smashes TV Records in US, Japan." http://www.fifa.com/womensworldcup/news/y=2015/m=7/news=world-cup-final-smashes-tv-records-in-us-japan-2661775.html.

Hall, M Ann 2003. "The Game of Choice: Girls' and Women's Soccer in Canada." *Soccer & Society* 4 (2-3): 30–46.

Hallmann, K. 2012. "Women's 2011 Football World Cup: The Impact of Perceived Images of Women's Soccer and the World Cup 2011 on Interest in Attending Matches." *Sport Management Review* 15: 33–42. doi:10.1016/j.smr.2011.05.002

Lopez, S. 1997. *Women on the Ball*. London: Scarlet Press.

Markovits, A. S. and S. L. Hellerman. 2003. "Women's Soccer in the United States: Yet Another American "Exceptionalism"." *Soccer & Society* 4 (2-3): 14–29.

The Football Association. 2015a. "Dads Urged to Support the FA's We Can Play Campaign." http://www.thefa.com/news/fawsl/2015/jun/the-fas-we-can-play-campaign-19062015.

The Football Association. 2015b. "Record Numbers Tune in to Support England's Women." http://www.thefa.com/news/england/womens/2015/jul/record-numbers-stay-up-to-cheer-on-lionesses-in-canada.

Williams, J. 2013. *A Beautiful Game: International Perspectives on Women's Football*. Oxford/New York: Berg.

Wright, J., and G. Clarke. 1999. "Sport, the Media and the Construction of Compulsory Heterosexuality: A Case Study of Women's Rugby Union." *International Review for the Sociology of Sport* 34 (3): 227–243.

'Trust me I am a Football Agent'. The discursive practices of the players' agents in (un)professional football

Seamus Kelly and Dikaia Chatziefstathiou

ABSTRACT

FIFA's decision to deregulate the industry is perhaps a reflection of the neoliberal influences surrounding the organization to let the agents govern themselves and deal with the wrongdoings of the alleged bribery, exploitation and trafficking of young players. However, it can also be seen as the organization's inefficiency to maintain the primacy of self-regulation and self-governance in matters such as agents' global leadership and regulation of practices. This paper, using qualitative data collected from players, agents and managers from professional football leagues in the UK and Ireland, aims to uncover the unethical, extremely complex and deceptive sides of the agents' industry. Two key issues are unpacked: (i) the alleged (un) ethical behaviour of football agents that provokes so much hostility in the football world; (ii) the power shift(s) from clubs and managers to agents and players and the implications these may have on the ethics of the business practices in football.

Introduction

Sport is an important venue for cultural interaction and the development of forms of moral consensus (about the rules, about how to behave in an appropriate manner etc.). Sport as a social phenomenon is neither inherently positive nor negative in its effects (Chatziefstathiou and Henry 2012). A tension exists between sport as an area of economic activity, subject to the rules and discourse of business and government regulation, and as an area of social, physical and moral self-development of civil society. Since the turn of the twenty-first century, sport has been increasingly experiencing its own deep crises, which undermines faith in sport's ability for self-regulation, and thus the legitimacy of its leading governing bodies, the International Olympic Committee (IOC) and *Fédération Internationale de Football Association* (FIFA).

Undoubtedly the most significant of these crises in Olympic terms was the Salt Lake City debacle in 1998 (Chatziefstathiou and Henry 2012). More than a decade later, in 2011, a governance crisis surfaced at FIFA. Doubts about the organization's ethical conduct in international football were previously raised by academics and in various media texts and outlets (see eg the book 'Badfellas' by Sugden and Tomlinson published in 2003; the book 'FOUL! The Secret World of FIFA: Bribes, Vote-Rigging and Ticket Scandals' followed by the BBC's Panorama documentary by Andrew Jennings in 2006). The investigations have led to guilty pleas or indictments of more than 40 football and marketing officials, while Sepp Blatter was banned from all football-related activities for eight years – later reduced to six – in December 2015. Although FIFA desperately tries to restore its reputation, more scandals may emerge from the ongoing investigations by French and Swiss prosecutors concerning the bidding process behind the 2018 and 2022 World Cups.

The above demonstrate that the world of sport, and particularly the world of football on which this paper focuses, is experiencing serious governance failures. While the public and media attention is largely fixated on the corruption scandals of high officials in international football, FIFA's decision in April 2015 to deregulate football agents, or intermediaries as they are now called, also raises concerns about its ability for self-regulation and governance. FIFA's introduction (2006) and subsequent updating (2008) of its regulations and legal frameworks governing the activity of agents in professional football has important implications on the inner workings of football. A key Foucauldian concept which could contribute to our understanding of these regulating processes is that of governmentality which refers to socio-political contexts where power is decentred and where members of a society play an active role in their own self-government as individuals and groups. This relationship is expressed in the semantic linking of 'governing' (*gouverner*) and modes of thought (*mentalité*) (Chatziefstathiou and Henry 2012). In this regard, FIFA's decision to deregulate the industry is perhaps a reflection of the neoliberal influences surrounding the organization to let the agents govern themselves and deal with the wrongdoings of the alleged bribery, exploitation and trafficking of young players. However, the deregulation of agents by FIFA can also be seen as the organization's inefficiency to maintain the primacy of self-regulation and self-governance in serious matters of the industry, such as agents' global leadership and regulation of practices.

This paper, using primary qualitative data collected from players, agents and managers from professional football leagues in the UK and Ireland, aims to uncover the unethical, extremely complex and deceptive sides of the agents' industry. By doing so, it aims to emphasize the need for gold standards of practice and leadership in the regulation of international football, which desperately needs to restore its integrity.

The role of agents in professional football

The role of an agent typically involves contract (re)negotiations for players and managers, scouting of players for clubs, managing players' and managers' image rights and providing financial, counselling and support services. However, their practices are often seen as secretive, mysterious and 'dark', driven by large monetary gains. Though most professional football managers will have an understanding of agent's involvement in player transfers, it is only through media exposure (BBC Panorama special investigations), numerous inquiries (eg Smith & Lord Stevens) and a number of high profile court cases that the general public's awareness of their questionable practices have been highlighted.

Football agents are not a new phenomenon for they played an important role in scouting and recruiting players on clubs behalf following the legalization of professional football in 1885 (Roderick 2006). The entrepreneurial agents of the early professional days tended to represent football clubs and not players and 'it was not until the mid-1970s that players began to turn to people "outside" the game for professional advice on contract and transfer negotiations' (Roderick 2006, 127). It was in the post-Bosman era of professional football, with greater value contracts on offer, as well as more out-of-contract footballers seeking to maximize their career potential, that there has been a significant increase in the number of players using agents in contract negotiations (Horne, Tomlinson, and Whannel 1999). For example, in 2001, there were '179 FIFA-registered agents in England, compared to 88 in France, 80 in Germany … and 54 in Italy' (Banks 2002, 167). By 2007, there were 325 registered agents in England (Poli 2010) and by 2015 this figure increased to 550 (Rossi, Semens, and Brocard 2016). In recent years, a number of solo agents have merged to form their own player representative companies or media companies that provide services traditionally associated with the solo agent. The escalation in the number of agents now operating in professional football can be attributed to three principal factors.

Firstly, from the mid-1990s, professional football 'underwent an unprecedented boom making the game more popular and affluent than at any other time in its long history' (Magee 2002, 218). Due to the clubs' improved financial status, many invested heavily in the acquisition of players in the hope of improving their on-field performance. This resulted in an upward spiralling of players' wages. For example, in the 2013–2014 season, the total wage costs for English Premier League clubs was £1.9 billion, while that of the Championship clubs exceeded £500 million. It is argued that the primary benefactors of football's increased wealth have been the players, a development that has not been lost on football agents (Szczepanik 2009). The fees that agents charge for their services is capped at 3% of the player's basic gross income or transfer compensation (FIFA 2014) having previously varied between 5 and 10% of the player's salary (Poli 2010). While detailed information relating to payments made by players to agents is difficult to attain, in recent years many clubs have made public any payments made by them to agents. For example, English Premier League clubs paid out £66 million in agent fees in the 2007–2008 season (Kelso 2009), £115 million in 2013–2014 season and by the end of the 2016–2017 season, this figure is estimated to exceed £174 million. In the 2003–2004 season Manchester United paid out £5.5 million to agents involved in the acquisition of nine players; this figure had grown to over £7.9 million in 2014 with Chelsea FC paying over £16.7 million in the same year. In particular, the Portuguese agency Gestifute received '£1.129 million for negotiating Cristiano Ronaldo's transfer to Manchester United' (Poli 2010, 203) while in 2009 Jorge Mendes reportedly earned £3.6 m of the £9 m Manchester United paid for Bebe, replacing the players former agent in the process (Conn 2012).

Secondly, and more importantly, Bosman's success in the European Court of Justice rendered the then transfer system illegal. The Bosman ruling opened up the British market for professional footballers beyond the UK, and players at the end of their contract were able to move freely across Europe. This ruling also provided English clubs with the opportunity to compete with European clubs for their top players. Football agents' close collaboration with club officials and managers has in many ways replaced the traditional role of the club scout in the recruitment of football talent (Magee 2002; Poli 2010). Crucially, many agents are now in a position to provide reliable information on the availability of playing talent globally which has considerably influenced the growth in the number of agents and reinforced their power in professional football in particular (Poli 2010). Moreover, as we shall see later, agents' access to privileged and sensitive information concerning players' salaries and their level of satisfaction at their current club considerably influences their power. The internationalization of the labour market for professional players and emergence of new talent pipelines in particular (Poli 2010), combined with the Bosman ruling, has had a perceptible effect of shifting power away from football clubs towards players and their agents (Whitehead 1998; O'Leary and Caiger 2000; Lonsdale 2004). Thus, players and their agents in particular are now in considerably stronger position to negotiate better contracts and more lucrative options both at home and abroad. This is an important point and will be explored in greater detail later.

Finally, it is important to identify the relative ease with which an individual can obtain an agent's licence. The process for becoming a licensed players' agent is relatively straight-forward[1] and begins with an application to the individuals national Football Association. Back in 2006, the English FA required every candidate to pass and agent examination and sign a 'Code of Professional Conduct' in which they 'pledge, without fail, to abide by the basic principles described therein when acting as a players' agent' (Football Association 2006, 13). In 2008, FIFA updated its regulations and introduced a legal framework, which governed the activity of agents in professional football (FIFA 2008). However, following FIFA's decision to deregulate agent's activities in 2015, applicants are no longer required to sit the player's agent examination, provide police verification letters or professional indemnity insurance (Jackson 2016). In theory, anybody in England can become an agent or intermediary provided they have an impeccable reputation, no criminal record, no conflicted interests and pay the English FA £500 in registration fees (Riach 2015; Jackson 2016). Each national football association is still required to draw up a list of all the licensed intermediaries in its territory and forward it to FIFA. Perhaps surprisingly, there are no pre-requisite educational qualifications or experience required to secure a registered agent licence.

The considerable influx of money into professional football combined with the expanded opportunities to recruit players, both at home and abroad, has had a direct effect on the increased number of agents now operating in professional football. Out-of-contract players in general and more successful players in particular provide lucrative opportunities for agents to get involved in football where they now occupy key roles in contract negotiations. Back in 1998, Maguire and Stead astutely argued that 'the appearance of agents as part of soccer's economic relations is likely to have a growing impact on the form and extent of international player movements, and the range and complexity of transfer activities are likely to increase' (61). More recently, attracted by the large commissions available and increased levels of power (Poli 2010), the agent has now become a central figure in the football transfer market (Cashmore 2000; Magee 2002). However, as we shall see later in this paper, professional football was 'unprepared for the increased involvement of agents, their business approach, and their rapid centralization in the transfer and contract negotiating processes' (Magee 2002, 230).

While non-academic studies have identified the unethical and in some cases illegal business practices adopted by some agents (Bower 2003; Scott 2007), a number of academic studies have identified the different types of agents and their role in professional football[2] (Magee 1998, 2002; Holt, Michie, and Oughton 2006; Roderick 2006; Siekmann et al. 2007; Poli 2010; Demazière and Jouvenet 2013). Moreover, few academic studies have conducted semi-structured tape-recorded interviews with agents in examining how they impact on the role of the professional football manager.

This paper will shed further light to the existing scholarship about the issues of ethics surrounding agents in professional football by unpacking two key issues: (i) the alleged (un) ethical behaviour of football agents that provokes so much hostility in the football world; (ii) the power shift(s) from clubs and managers to agents and players and the implications these may have on the ethics of football business.

Methodology

This paper examines qualitative data collected over 10 years in two distinct stages. Stage one of the data collection occurred between 2004 and 2006 and involved semi-structured tape-recorded interviews with twenty-five players, five agents and twenty managers. The interviewees were players and managers who were either currently, or who had previously been, employed as professionals within the league structure in England and/or Ireland. The playing and/or managing careers of those interviewed lay between the extremes of outstanding professional success and more modest success. Some of the interviewees had played or managed at international level, while others had spent their entire careers in the lower leagues. More specifically, of the 25 players who were interviewed, 18 had experience as full-time professionals with clubs in the English Premier League. Three players had played at full international and eight at Under-21 level. Of the twenty managers who were interviewed, eight had managed clubs in England and three of these were managing English clubs at the time of the interviews. Several interviewees had managed clubs in both England and Ireland and two interviewees had managed a full senior international side. In 2015, stage two of the data collection involved semi-structured interviews with four players with experience of the academy structure at English Premier League and Championship teams. This sample of interviewees was a convenience sample, based on the personal contacts of the first author, and this sample was then expanded on a 'snowball' basis, with interviewees being asked after the interview if they knew of other players or managers whom they thought might be prepared to be interviewed. At the outset of each interview, interviewees were given an assurance of anonymity. This was designed to reduce interviewees' anxieties about discussing former or current managers and/or players. The data collected suggest that interviewees felt sufficiently confident to be relatively open and forthcoming in describing their own experiences in, and of, professional soccer in the UK.

What we tried to unpack in the data analysis process were the discursive practices of the football agents as being interpreted and witnessed from the agents themselves but also from other key persons in the industry such as players and managers. In Foucauldian terms 'discursive practice' is the process through which dominant reality comes into being. Such process involves the construction and reflection of social realities through actions that conjures up identity, ideology, belief and questions of power. Thus, the discourses of our interviewees can constitute our 'knowledge' about what is 'true' within the world of agents, and the world of football more broadly. We accept that knowledge is formed in the 'inter-action of plural and contingent practices within different sites, each of which involves the material and the symbolic' (Bacchi and Bonham 2014, 174). The term 'discursive practice/s' describes those practices of knowledge formation by focusing on how specific knowledges ('discourses') operate and the work they do (Bacchi and Bonham 2014). Our data helped us to form such knowledge about the complex dynamics of power, which are negotiated, and in constant flux within what seems to be a rather unregulated environment. Two key issues emerged from the data analysis process: (i) there is a public and industry hostility against the football agents, mainly attributed to their alleged unethical behaviour and practices; (ii) the power shift(s) from clubs and managers to the agents and players – mainly as a result of the internationalization of football and of the Bosman ruling – has enhanced the agents' role with serious implications in the industry. These points are discussed next in more detail.

Hostility towards agents

Because of the proliferation of agents in professional football, there is a widely held view by many people in professional football that agents are damaging the game. Napoli's owner, Aurelio de Laurentiis, has described them as the 'cancer of our world', further stating that football 'does not need them' (BBC 2016). Data gathered from managers, players, and surprisingly, even from some agents, echo this hostility towards football agents and their business practices in particular. Many of the football managers interviewed described agents as 'parasites' and 'con-men', while players viewed them as 'scumbags' and 'cowboys'. During the course of an interview, one manager with considerable experience in Ireland and England became very animated when the issue of agents arose. Shifting uncomfortably in his seat, he described agents in the following terms:

> They are a disaster, an absolute disaster. I just have no time for them, and I've dealt with quite a few. I've dealt with so many of them in England, not so many here [Ireland]. I've met many of them in England, and I have yet to meet a good one, a genuine one. They're parasites.

Several managers expressed the view that players do not need agents. One manager said: 'Now I am not saying that a player shouldn't be represented, but I feel that their union should represent them. There are representatives in the union and they are qualified to do so'. In this regard, the English FA argues against the need for players to employ agents, saying that rather than being 'ripped off', players would be better advised to use their own union, the Professional Footballers' Association (PFA), which was better equipped and cheaper as an option (Roderick 2000; Magee 2002). The data reported in this research reinforce the views held by the English FA that 'players do not need agents' (O'Leary and Caiger 2000, 272). The following two examples from managers with experience in the English Premier League were typical of managers' views:

> To be honest with you the view I'd have is, I wouldn't have a problem, if a player has an agent as I said, but I think they are foolish to have agents. That's my view.

> They are in the game, they are part of the game and they have to be dealt with. You have to deal with them professionally. The nature of the game is that everyone knows everyone so there is possibly not a need, from a manager's point of view, to go through an agent. From a players point of view he is protecting his own interest during negotiations, maybe to strengthen his negotiations, then I don't have a problem.

Roderick (2003, 272) suggested that agents 'close association with their clients, in terms of negotiating on their behalf and often in their absence, leaves open the possibility for shady manoeuvring in relation to the way in which the players' agents conduct their business'. A recurring theme that emerged from the interviews with managers concerned their distrustful attitudes towards agents. For example, one former English Championship League manager said:

> I've used xxxx [agent's name] a few times. Yeah, you come across them from time to time. I find that if there is an agent involved there is a motive. And I'm not saying that is negative or positive, but there is a motive there in some way. I've taken me chances with them and I've dealt with them and some of them are absolute chancers and I've signed a few dummies in my time.

Despite such hostility towards agents, developing personal contact networks with agents considered as 'trustworthy' is viewed as crucial in order to operate within 'the player transfer and representation business' (Poli and Rossi 2012, 60). More specifically, current agent and former Danish international Mikkel Beck stated:

> despite all the money that is involved, and how much importance people place on it, the only way you can be successful is to build up trust with your client. I have always had excellent relationships with my client's families. (Evans 2013, 37)

A similar theme emerged from the interviews with players, who identified the importance of securing the services of an agent with whom they could trust. The following two examples from players with experience in the English Premier League were typical of players' views:

> I mean there is always going to be bad cloud hanging over agents. But I think if you can get the right one and someone who is legitimate, from a player's point of view, like, its great … it takes so much pressure off you. I think the trust factor is very important.

Implicit in the above data is the importance of trust between players and agents (Demazière and Jouvenet 2013). However, the data collected from players and managers suggest that agents have acquired a poor reputation which may, in part, impact on their ability to do business in professional football. In this regard, some clubs and managers refuse to deal with certain agents. This point was developed further during the course of an interview with an agent who was working with a prominent England-based sports agency company:

> Yeah, like there are a lot of managers who will not deal with certain agents. I mean that's why in this business it's all about reputation and trust. If you're working in a company … the company's reputation is so important, and you would never do anything to jeopardise that. I mean not even one thing wrong, because word spreads very quickly. You know it takes a long time to build up a good reputation, and it's very easy to get a bad reputation.

In the context of player contract (re)negotiations there is some evidence to suggest that it is not just agents who have acquired poor reputations. Some managers adopt tactics such as 'tapping up' in their attempts to sign prospective players. All of the agents interviewed were asked to describe their experiences of negotiating player contracts with managers. One licensed agent described some of the difficulties that he had experienced when negotiating with managers on their players behalf.

> Agent: Yeah, sometimes it can be difficult. Yeah, well actually it is a nightmare at times. I mean, people lie through their teeth to get players, like blatant lies.

> Interviewer: Really, like who?

> Agent: Managers. Yeah, I mean … like you are talking to managers and they are blatantly lying to you and you know it. Like they are trying to play cute and be dull, it's just unbelievable what is going on.

Currently there are many agents operating in professional football and considering the level of competition amongst agents, acquiring a client base is a crucial strategy for agents. The PFA representative Mick McGuire noted that 'there are a few top agents who have grabbed the market and … eighty per cent are fighting over the crumbs' (Magee 2002, 232). This strong competition between agents for players may encourage some agents to engage in illegal or ethically debatable practices (Poli 2010). Implicit in the above data, and developed further in the next section, is how professional football has often been described as an industry characterized by endemic distrust (Roderick 2006), mainly due to the unethical and questionable practices adopted by some agents.

Unethical and questionable practices

Numerous concerns have been publicly expressed in relation to the alleged unethical and illegal practices adopted by some agents. For example, serious ethical concerns have been raised about the treatment of young African playing talent during the 1990s by unscrupulous agents and speculators (Broere and van der Drift 1997; Darby, Akindes, and Kirwin 2007) who 'recognized in the trade in African talent an opportunity for personal financial gain' (Darby, Akindes, and Kirwin 2007, 147). Illegal payments have long been a feature of English football since its professionalization in 1885. The testimonies collected by Taylor and Ward (1995) suggested that under-the-counter payments, or 'backhanders', to players were common ways of circumventing the wage restrictions in the 1950s. Evidence suggests that questionable practices and illegal payments are still common practice in professional football. For example, one licensed agent, who was at the time of the interview working for a leading UK-based sports agency company, described the nature of the player representation industry and the level of competition that exists within the industry. In particular, he described some of the debatable practices adopted by some agents:

You know there are a lot of people in the business who are backstabbers and who lie. Like some people would say things about the [agents] company, or me, which aren't true, you know.In addition, one former English Premier League manager described, during the course of an interview, the role of agents in professional football as 'a load of bollocks, a shitty business, they are greedy and are full of f***** hookery'. One recurring theme from the data gathered from players, managers and agents concerned how 'backhanders' and 'dodgy' payments are still common aspects of professional football. During the course of an interview with a former manager discussions focussed on how he dealt with such behaviour. When probed further about how he managed in that kind of an industry and in such an environment, he stated:

Manager: [Leaning forward in his chair and pointing his finger at me] Well I'll tell you how you manage, and how you can stay the distance. You've got to be so street wise, and you've got to be so f***** sharp, because it's stinking, it's absolutely stinking.

In professional football, it is not unusual for managers and/or players to be contacted by agents to broker or facilitate a deal. Moreover, the manager's comment above reveals the questionable tactics some agents will adopt in facilitating a move for their player and the nature of the industry in particular. In this regard, the court case in 2007 involving Stewart Downing shed light on the how some agents may abuse the player–agent relationship and siphon money from player's personal bank accounts (Collins 2011). In not too dissimilar manner, a number of players identified that they were distrustful of agents. Several players described situations where they had been 'messed around' by agents. For example, one former senior international player with considerable English Premiership experience described a situation where a fellow player received a massive sum of money when he signed for a particular club. However, it transpired that the money he received from the agent was only a loan to the player. He said:

> There was this one player, who didn't realise and who got a massive amount of money, I think it was £50,000 and he had to pay it back to xxxx [the agent]. The agent said to the player: 'Like you didn't read the small print, that the money was only a loan'. You know that's the kind of stuff that goes on and you know it's an absolute disgrace, so you just have to be very very careful.

Given the levels of hostility and distrust towards agents, one obvious question arises: why are agents so widely utilized by managers and players? The following section attempts to answer this question.

Shifting balances of power and conflicts of interests

Stead (1999, 24) has argued that 'player power has increased disproportionately at the very highest levels of English football' while Magee (2002) highlighted the difficulties of working with agents and the increased power which they now possess in relation to clubs. Therefore, and despite doubts over their motives and actions, it has become almost impossible for managers not to deal with certain agents. This is because failure to do so may result in a manager not securing the services of particular players whom he wishes to sign.

Based on the data collected, there is considerable evidence to illustrate the power of some agents in general and football clubs' dependence on agents in particular. For example, one former English Premier League player described how the arrival of a prominent international player at the club was mired in scandal. Two weeks after the arrival of the international star, a second unknown player was signed. The player described how his fellow players at the club responded to this second signing with considerable scepticism. The player, raising his eyes to the ceiling stated that, 'all hell broke loose' when it transpired that the second player had been signed simply to provide a large fee for the agent. Raising his voice the player said, 'It was a f****** disgrace' and explained exactly what had happened:

> What happened was that the international player wanted to use his own agent, while the club insisted that the player use the Premiership club's agent. When the player and his agent refused the club's request, the club were forced to use the player's agent. When the club's agent found out about this he was furious and threatened to withdraw his services from the club. To sort the whole thing out, the club asked the agent to select a player (from his portfolio of players, who had signed up with the agent), which the club would sign and the agent would then get his commission (having lost out on his commission from the international players deal). The players at the club went ballistic that this player had been signed, even though no one had any knowledge of the player. I mean, I '*BURST MY B*******'* to get a full contract … and this chap just gets one off the back of that'. It was a f****** joke.

Implicit in the above players' comments is the power some agents have assumed and one important point. Firstly, this club's insistence that the player use the club's agent breached the then English FA's regulations governing agent practices. More specifically, conflicts of interest are prohibited and occur when an agent represents both a player and a club. The issue arises where one has a duty to act in the best interests of two or more different parties and the duties conflict, or there is a risk that they may conflict. Governance issues concerning dubious practices such as conflicts of interest, 'dual representation' (Conn 2016), referred to as 'duality' (Booker 2016), are commonly reported by the media (Taylor 2007; Conn 2016). This point was particularly evident when questions were raised following the arrival of Jose Mourinho to Chelsea in 2004. In particular, the English FA permitted the agent, Jorge Mendes, to act for both the club and players in the same transfer involving a number of Mourinhos' former Porto players. However, despite an apparent breach of FIFA regulations these transfers were allowed by the English FA at the time (Conn 2012). It seems that dual representation may be allowed if both sides agree to waive any concern that the agent may have a conflict of interest (Conn 2016).

In recent years, players in general and those players who are considered more valuable in terms of their playing talent in particular have been able to exercise greater muscle in contract negotiations with their manager. However, the level of power that players possess varies considerably. By definition, the improved ability to sell one's labour applies most to those players who are in great demand. Post-Bosman, clubs began to offer improved terms to players under contract to keep them at the clubs. As a result, players are now able to use the threat of seeing out a contract and taking a transfer-free move as a lever to negotiate improved terms in their existing contract. In comparison to their pre-Bosman predecessors, this is a relatively powerful position for players, especially the top ones, as clubs cannot afford to lose a player without a transfer reimbursement. The removal of transfer fees and the potential severance notice has allowed players and their agents greater bargaining power to demand increased wages without the necessary contract commitment that was a feature of the pre-Bosman transfer system.[3] The increased power which players have assumed was a recurring theme in the interviews with players, managers and agents. More specifically, one former English Championship player stated:

> Players now can talk to other clubs long before their contracts end so if they go into negotiations they can say that this club has offered this. I've got this, that and you know that they [the clubs] must basically match it. And also with more agents in the game now the players are getting better deals. The agents are looking after the players. When they look after the players as best they can it puts the players in a powerful position.

Similarly, one UK-based licensed agent described the shifting balance of power towards players:

> I think in the last ten years a lot of the power has shifted towards the player's side of things, with the Bosman and different things like that, you know where before, I think clubs had so much power over players and now it's kind of turned full circle. Clubs nowadays are afraid of players going on a free [transfer] and you have the ridiculous wages that they are looking for and transfer fees are crazy, like you can see it now that clubs are struggling big time ... but I think definitely that the players have more power at the moment.

It seems that agents have exploited this shift in players' bargaining power. Magee has argued (2002, 230) that 'even though the player has gained significant control ... it is the agent who ultimately controls and potentially exploits the player'. More recently, David Conn has identified how the practice of 'switching' agents seems to suggest a further attempt to shift power towards agents in general and club appointed agents in particular (Conn 2016). Moreover, the presence of 'multiple agency agreements' (Jackson 2016) between agents and players reflects not only a lack of governance mechanisms but players', and their families in particular, preference for securing the 'best deal' on offer. What this means is that the more 'marketable players' can now secure the best deal on offer. Moreover, it is not uncommon for the more powerful agents to undermine lucrative deals, with the players' registered agent receiving a 'facilitators' fee. In this regard, it is not uncommon for players' family members to receive 'gifts' in an effort to secure their services. However, as discussed earlier, some managers may also attempt to open a rift between the player and the agent by challenging the abilities of an agent during negotiations. This point is borne out by O'Leary and Caiger

(2000) who describe an interview between a manager, a player and the player's agent. The manager said:

> We try to bypass agents. We signed a player. He had his agent present at the negotiation. The agent asked for an impossible salary. The agent wanted £15,000 and £500 per week. The player was on £450 per week and was not in the first team. The agent said: 'My client won't accept the deal'. I said to the player   'where did you get this prat from – we want your contract, why don't you tell him to go?' The agent protested. I said to the player: 'do you want to sign for us or not?' He said 'Yes' and told the agent to leave.

This manager's reluctance to deal with agents may be in part a reflection of managers' frustration 'at the changing balance of contractual power' (O'Leary and Caiger 2000, 273). Roderick (2003, 228) has suggested that the relative power which players possess 'may depend on factors such as their age and the work-related reputations they develop'. Magee (1998) developed a useful typology and suggested players could be categorized into three broad groupings. The first group of players, 'the exploiters', is those players whose talent is sought after. Secondly, 'the exploited', are those players who have relatively few choices in terms of career options and choice of club and have relatively little power to determine their future. If one imagines these two groupings of players at the extremes of a continuum, then players who are referred to as 'the marketable' occupy middle positions. The 'marketable' are players who are viewed as club assets and may be sold in order to generate capital and to relieve financial pressures. Such 'marketable' players have a value which managers may be able to exploit for their own interests. As Magee (1998) suggests, the 'exploiters' are powerful in the sense that they are in a strong bargaining position, while 'the exploited' would have considerably less power. It is clear that these three ideal types of players must be considered in relational terms for players are never in, or out of, full control. More specifically, it is a question of power ratios or balances, and over time players' positions on this continuum will change. For example, players grow older, or suffer serious injury while coaches or managers opinions of their playing performance may also change. Thus, the degree of power which players and their agents have in relation to a club or manager depends largely on the players' position on this continuum. One registered agent was questioned whether he viewed players possessing more power in recent years.

> I think the players have a lot of power now. I think it comes down to how well you are doing how much power you have individually. But if you are not doing it on the pitch there are not too many people looking for you. So basically you have to be doing it on the pitch to have the power. You have to be putting in the performances you know.

Agents, managers and players are all bound up in a complex process and each must take into account the actions of the others. The people who occupy central positions within these networks of relations have power insofar as they are less dependent on specific others, while those others are more dependent on them. Managers, for instance, rely on the levels of performance achieved by their players and this in turn can be a means by which players can exercise a degree of power over their employers. Conversely, club managers can utilize the threat of rejection as a means of exercising power over prospective players or omitting current players from the playing squad. Thus, an examination of the dynamic balances of power among those involved in the network of relations within professional football – such as players, managers and agents – is essential to understand adequately the role which each plays.

These balances of power form an integral element of all human relationships. To put it at its simplest, 'when one person, or a group of persons lacks something which another person or group has the power to withhold, the latter has a function for the former' (Mennell and Goudsblom 1998, 119). Therefore, people or groups, which have functions for each other, exercise constraints over each other. Their potential for withholding from each other what the other requires is usually uneven, which means that the constraining power of one side is greater than that of the other. In the overall nexus of interdependencies, individuals may question another individual's power of constraint, or their 'potential for withholding'. These in effect are trials of strength between two parties. At the root of these trials of strength are usually problems such as: 'Who, therefore, has to submit or adapt himself more to the others demands?' (Mennell and Goudsblom 1998, 120). Put simply, who can put more pressure on whom? Agents, it can be argued, have greater power, or power ratios, when representing a player who, in Magee's (1998) terms, is considered an 'exploiter'. That is not to say that the 'exploited' possess no power, but their power is more limited. These power resources and relative strengths are constantly tested. Each side tries to weaken the other by a variety of means, and both sides are involved in a continuous process of interweaving actions with each other and with other groups. The sequence of moves on either side can only be understood and explained in terms of the immanent dynamics of their interdependence.

Conclusion

If we accept that the discourses of our interviewees can constitute our 'knowledge' about what is 'true' within the world of agents, and the world of football more broadly, our data have further reinforced the general perception that the agents' industry is unethical, extremely complex and deceptive. The dominant reality, which has been shaped through the discursive practices of the key stakeholders, is one of a 'messy' business. FIFA decided in 2015 to pass the regulation of the agents' industry to individual national associations, and 'the result has seen a huge disparity in standards between different jurisdictions' (Conliff 2017). The natural question is whether key stakeholders such as FIFA, UEFA and national football associations could regulate the governance of the game. Historically, in terms of agent regulations, one of the major problems concerned the discrepancy between FIFA and national governing bodies' regulations (Siekmann et al. 2007). In relation to this, Giambattista Rossi, coauthor of *Sports Agents and Labour Markets*, believes that European football's governing body failed to show leadership in April 2015.

> I blame UEFA. They should have stood up and said: 'We are the best example of football in the world – in terms of governance, transparency, whatever – so let's prepare a proposal to regulate agents at least at European level. And then, in China, Brazil, wherever, they [will] want to follow us because the main turnover of transfers is in Europe.' (Jackson 2016)

As mentioned earlier in this paper, FIFA's decision to deregulate the industry could be interpreted as a reflection of neoliberal influences. This can be related to the notion of governmentality where power is de-centred and the members of society play an active role in their own self-government, eg as assumed in neoliberalism. Such active role delegates regulation to individuals who are regulated from 'inside' in a process of self-government and self-regulation (Foucault 1991). The knowledge that is produced within this frame of neoliberalist governmentality allows for the construction of auto-regulated or auto-cor-recting selves. Indeed, FIFA's absence from maintaining the primacy of self-regulation and self-governance in relation to global leadership and regulation of practices has led individuals to organize and 'govern' themselves through initiatives such as campaigns for instigating an effective system of self-regulation, eg through SOFIA, the Society of Football Intermediaries and Agents.

However, FIFA's decision also reflects its inability to deal with the agents' complex industry, especially at a time when the scandals of its senior officials were just far too many to manage. FIFA had to 'pick up her fights' and regulating the agents' industry was beyond it now. As a result, agents are still holding a considerably powerful position in professional football, while the lack of quality control over the granting of agent licences continues to raise issues concerning the ethical and legal aspects of their behaviour.

Notes

1. Prior to deregulation, in order to undertake the work of a players' agent, an individual must be one of the following: a licensed players' agent; a solicitor or barrister in possession of a current practicing certificate; the parent, spouse or sibling of the particular player in question. Players may still represent themselves.
2. There are at least four types of agent operating in professional football. Firstly, the most popular type is the solo agent. These are licensed agents who deal mainly with transfers and contracts. Secondly, the sports agency which provides a wider support service beyond contract negotiations and also has an agents licence. Thirdly, the solicitor who provides legal services and may not have an agents licence. Finally, the promotions agency, which provides advice on career management and promotion opportunities but has no agents licence.
3. Under FIFA regulations, a player is allowed to commence negotiations with other clubs six months from the end of a contract. From a player's perspective it seems only reasonable that a player be allowed to negotiate during, what is in effect, his notice period. However players who have already negotiated and signed contracts with rival clubs for the next season are placed in a position where, should the teams meet, a conflict of interest may arise.

Disclosure statement

No potential conflict of interest was reported by the authors.

References

Bacchi, C., and J. Bonham. 2014. "Reclaiming Discursive Practices as an Analytic Focus: Political Implications." *Foucault Studies* 17: 173–192.

Banks, S. 2002. *Going Down: Football in Crisis, How the Game Went from Boom to Bust*. London: Mainstream.

BBC. 2016. "Aurelio De Laurentiis: Agents 'a Cancer' on Football and Not Needed," October 5. Accessed May 5, 2017. http://www.bbc.co.uk/sport/football/37570186

Booker, J. 2016. "Corrupt Behavior has Become Endemic in Footballs Culture." *Guardian*, September 29.

Bower, T. 2003. *Broken Dreams: Vanity, Greed and the Souring of Football*. London: Simon & Schuster.

Broere, M., and R. van der Drift. 1997. *Football Africa!* Oxford: WorldView.

Cashmore, E. 2000. *Making Sense of Sports*. London: Routledge.

Chatziefstathiou, D., and I. P. Henry. 2012. *Discourses of Olympism. From the Sorbonne 1894 to London 2012*. Cambridge: Palgrave.

Collins, N. 2011. "Football Agent 'Siphoned Hundreds of Thousands' from England Star's Account." *Telegraph*, March 8.

Conliff, P. 2017. "State of Play: Time to Ensure Regulation of Agents." *The Irish Times*, April 28.

Conn, D. 2012. "Portuguese Police to Question Manchester United over Bébé Transfer." *Guardian*, May 10.

Conn, D. 2016. "Chelsea and Watford Face Questions over Agent Links." *Guardian*, December 14.

Darby, P., G. Akindes, and M. Kirwin. 2007. "Football Academies and the Migration of African Football Labor to Europe." *Journal of Sport and Social Issues* 31: 143–161. doi:10.1177/0193723507300481

Demazière, D., and M. Jouvenet. 2013. "The Market Work of Football Agents and the Manifold Valorizations of Professional Football Players. Economic Sociology." *The European Electronic Newsletter* 15 (1): 29–40.

Evans, O. 2013. "Secret Agents." *Sport Business International* 195 (11): 36–37.

FIFA. 2006. *Players' Agent Regulations*. Zurich: FIFA.

FIFA. 2008. *Players' Agent Regulations*. Zurich: FIFA.

FIFA. 2014. *Regulations on Working with Intermediaries*. Zurich: FIFA.

Football Association. 2006. *The Football Association: Football Agent Regulations*. London: FA.

Foucault, M. 1991. "Governmentality." Translated by Rosi Braidotti and Revised by Colin Gordon. In *The Foucault Effect: Studies in Governmentality*, edited by Graham Burchell, Colin Gordon, and Peter Miller, 87–104. Chicago, IL: University of Chicago Press.

Holt, M., J. Michie, and C. Oughton. 2006. *The Role and Regulation of Agents in Football*. London: The Sports Nexus.

Horne, J., A. Tomlinson, and G. Whannel. 1999. *Understanding Sport: An Introduction to the Sociological and Cultural Analysis of Sport*. London: Spon.

Jackson, J. 2016. "Football Insiders Claim World Game is 'Endemically Corrupt' in Player Transfers." *Guardian*, October 9.

Kelso, P. 2009. "Premier League Wages Soar as Agents Paid £66 Million." *Daily Telegraph*, June 4.

Lonsdale, C. 2004. "Player Power: Capturing Value in the English Football Supply Network." *Supply Chain Management: An International Journal*. 9 (5): 383–391. doi:10.1108/13598540410560766

Magee, J. D. 1998. "International Labour Migration in English League Football." Unpublished PhD thesis, University of Brighton.

Magee, J. 2002. "Shifting Balances of Power in the New Football Economy." In *Power Games: Theory and Method for the Critical Sociology of Sport*, edited by J. Sugden and A. Tomlinson, 216–239. London: Routledge.

Mennell, S., and J. Goudsblom. 1998. *Norbert Elias on Civilisation, Power and Knowledge*. Edited with an Introduction by Stephen Mennell and Johan Goudsblom. London: The University of Chicago Press.

O'Leary, J., and A. Caiger. 2000. "Shifting Power and Control in English Football." *New Zealand Journal of Industrial Relations* 25 (3): 259–275.

Poli, R. 2010. "Agents and Intermediaries." In *Managing Football*, edited by Sean Hamil and Simon Chadwick, 201–216. Oxford: Elsevier.

Poli, R., and G. Rossi. 2012. *Football Agents in the Biggest Five European Football Markets an Empirical Research Report*. Neuchâtel: Centre International d'Etude du Sport.

Riach, J. 2015. *Football Agents Fear 'Wild West' as FIFA Reforms Seek to Cap Fees*. The Guardian, March 31.

Roderick, M. 2000. *The Role of Agents in Professional Football. In Singer & Friedlander Review 2000–2001 Season*. London: Singer and Friedlander.

Roderick, M. 2003. "A Labour of Love: Careers in Professional Football." Unpublished PhD thesis, University of Leicester.

Roderick, M. 2006. *The Work of Professional Football: A Labour of Love*. London: Routledge.

Rossi, G., A. Semens, and J. F. Brocard. 2016. *Sports Agents and Labour Markets: Evidence from World Football*. London: Routledge.

Scott, M. 2007. "Stevens Bung Inquiry Reports 'Serious Breaches.'" *Guardian*, June 8.

Siekmann, R., R. Parrish, R. B. Martins, and J. Soek. 2007. *Players' Agents Worldwide*. Cambridge: Cambridge University Press. doi:10.1007/978-90-6704-551-3

Stead, D. 1999. "The 'Bosman Legacy': Some Reflections on the Bosman Case's Impact on English Football." In *Singer and Friedlander Review, 1998-99 Season*, edited by P. Murphy, 23–26. Leicester: University of Leicester.

Sugden, J., and A. Tomlinson. 2003. *Badfellas: FIFA Family at War*. Edinburgh: Mainstream.

Szczepanik, N. 2009. "Players the Winners as Football Bucks Trend." *The Times*, June 4.

Taylor, A. 2007. "Agent Denies Conflict of Interest over Megson." *Guardian*, October 26.

Taylor, R., and A. Ward. 1995. *Kicking and Screaming: An Oral History of Football in England*. London: Robson Books.

Whitehead, M. 1998. "Bosmania! Player Power Gone Mad?" *Sports Law Administration & Practice* 5 (6): 1–6.

Motorsport volunteerism: a form of social contract?

David Hassan and Chris Harding

ABSTRACT

The field of sports volunteerism has received considerable attention over recent years. It is increasingly evident that many national and transnational governing bodies of sport accept that the sustainability of their events remains conditional upon volunteers who are willing to offer their skills and labour free of charge. Fortunately, something of a resurgence within volunteerism, especially around sporting events, appears to be taking hold, albeit largely within the Global North, and so, it is appropriate to consider whether this may be explained with reference to the under-examined field of social contract theory. This therefore is the primary aim of this article, which draws specific attention to this phenomenon within motorsport. It concludes that there is indeed considerable evidence that motorsport volunteers are encouraged to provide their services in a manner consistent with some form of contractual obligation, and thus, in a wider sense, these conclusions offer valuable insights for other sporting bodies regarding their volunteer recruitment and retention strategies in the time ahead.

Introduction

A broadly accepted definition of 'volunteerism' remains somewhat elusive. This is due largely to the absence of agreement concerning what is understood by the act of volunteering. A lack of consensus, specifically around philosophical, cultural and ethical interpretations of the work of volunteers, further adds to these complexities. Given such difficulties, it is typical to rely upon open-ended definitions of volunteerism, such as that offered by the UN General Assembly, which defines the practice as reflecting: 'A wide range of activities, including traditional forms of mutual aid and self-help, formal service delivery and other forms of civic participation undertaken of free will for the general public good and where monetary reward is not the principal motivating factor' (The Executive Board of the United Nations Development Programme, 2013, 54). That said, extant literature also confirms that, rather than pursuing one single definition, we should think of volunteerism as reflecting a number of agreed characteristics, such as those described below by the International Labour Organisation:

- An activity or work completed in-kind, carried out by people;
- Performed willingly by free choice independent of external forces and without payment;

- Done to promote a cause or help someone outside of the volunteer's household or immediate family; and/or
- Formally performed, through an organization or informally on an individual basis.

Thus, in a general sense, volunteerism can be thought of as the provision of a service agreed to under personal freedom of choice for no expected monetary gain. Notwithstanding this, the wider ethical issues surrounding the treatment and levels of expectations around the contributions made by volunteers, particularly in certain sporting settings, appear to be growing in a variety of ways.

The role of volunteerism in sport

Volunteers are accepted as being a core component of sports delivery at all levels of the industry (Green and Chalip 1998; Giannoulakis, Wang, and Gray 2008). It is generally understood that the majority of sporting organizations would be unable to function effectively were not for the assistance of volunteers (Auld and Cuskelly 2001).

When sports volunteerism is discussed in the public realm, an association with large-scale events, such as the Summer Olympic Games, is typically formed. In many respects, this is a valid position, as these spectacles attract volunteers in multiple of thousands, and indeed, it is the contribution of the volunteers themselves that is often the key message to emerge from such mega-sport events. The capacity of major events to attract large numbers of volunteers is also noteworthy. The 2010 Winter Olympic Games in Vancouver, Canada, drew a volunteer body of some 18,500 individuals (Vancouver Olympics Commission 2010), whilst in the same year almost 68,000 people applied to volunteer at the FIFA World Cup in South Africa, from which 18,000 were ultimately recruited (CNN Corporation 2010).

However, volunteers are not only found at prestigious international sporting events. At a national and regional level, such individuals perform equally significant roles. For example, the Special Olympics International movement was assisted by over 306,000 volunteer coaches and an additional 800,000 voluntary youth assistants during 2011 alone, a remarkable contribution of 'in-kind' labour. Even at a community level, volunteers make important contributions, which are admittedly sometimes not always appreciated by those who benefit from their input.

An appropriate example of this can be established in Europe, specifically Ireland, where volunteers perform a crucial function in the organization, promotion and management of Gaelic Games under the administration of the indigenous sporting body, the Gaelic Athletic Association (GAA). These sporting activities are very much at the heart of local communities in Ireland with the majority of coaches, administrators and organizers employed in a voluntary capacity. Such assistants offer their time for the enjoyment of the sport by others, the development of a strong regional identity and the creation of sporting opportunities, in particular, for young people from their surrounding locality. Without the contribution of these volunteers, it is unlikely that this sporting body could continue to exist from one generation to the next, as it has successfully done so for the past 133 years.

The demographic profile of sports volunteers and international presence

With volunteering being understood as critical to the success of the sports industry, it is surprising that only a small number of countries actually record data around volunteering levels. Within those countries that do, it is clear that sports volunteerism remains a common and popular activity. For example, in 2010, almost 2 million adults in England contributed at least one hour per week to voluntary sporting activities, more than in any other sector. In New Zealand, almost 830,000 individuals volunteered in sport in 2007, approximately 25.3% of the entire population of that country (Dalziel 2011). In Australia, sports volunteers are recognized as being a highly important component of national public policy reflected in the numbers of volunteers committed to Australian sport (Zakus, Skinner, and Edwards 2009). For example, in 2006, over 1.7 million Australian citizens volunteered in sport and often in more than one role (Australian Bureau of Statistics 2012). Canada also possesses relatively high levels of sports volunteers, with 18% of the total volunteers in the country offering their services to this realm during 2009 – the equivalent of an additional workforce of 262,000 full-time paid employees (Statistics Canada 2010).

Studies have been conducted that aim to capture the demographic profile of those individuals who volunteer. A key finding of such studies reveals that these individuals possess a high level of educational attainment as well as comfortable levels of disposable income. However, this finding is often only apparent amongst those volunteers aged 35 years or over (Lunn and Layte 2009). In contrast, younger volunteers typically emerge from lower socio-economic backgrounds, which is an interesting development in its own right. In an informative study, again from Ireland and conducted in 2005, it was found that sports volunteerism was commonplace amongst professionals, with 20% of those surveyed holding roles at middle-management levels. This study also confirmed how sports volunteerism is more prevalent amongst the self-employed and somewhat less so amongst those who are retired or seeking work. An interesting correlation was also established, albeit only in certain cases, between individuals who volunteer in sports and those with a registered disability, particularly amongst those older than 44 years of age (Irish Sport Council 2007).

These findings are broadly in line with other studies conducted on this subject. In research undertaken by Sports England in 2003, it was noted that a relatively even percentage of volunteers could be identified within each social demographic. However, the highest percentages of volunteers (8.5%) were located in the 16- to 19-year-old category, as well as the 35- to 44-year-old demographic. A notable decrease was again evident in over 65-year-old demographic (2.9%). One aspect of this study, which represents something of a departure from otherwise similar work conducted in this field, is that twice the numbers of volunteers were male (67%) as opposed to (33%) female (Sports Volunteers in England). In other similar studies, however, such a marked disparity between genders was not as clear (Dalziel 2011). This particular study also found that 54% of sports volunteers surveyed were classified as being 'moderately to highly educated' and, again, representative of an elevated socio-economic background generally.

Motivations for volunteerism in sport

There is a consensus concerning the primary motivational factors that give rise to volunteerism in sport. One of the main reasons relates to one's own personal and professional development (Sports Volunteers in England 2002 2003). Many volunteers offer their time and services with the broad intention of acquiring new skills, knowledge and, in some cases, valuable work experience. The opportunity to improve core competencies in this way can be difficult to overlook in highly competitive job markets and, particularly so, in situations where an individual has accrued otherwise limited work experience.

A willingness and desire to develop and better one's own community represent another important motivational component of volunteer activity. Many individuals who do volunteer report a heightened sense of obligation and attachment to their community, and in such cultures, volunteerism is understood as being an integral part of civic society (Omoto and Snyder 2002). This kind of activity remains very much altruistic in nature, with satisfaction derived from 'giving something back' to the community or in assisting a particular sports institution, which may retain personal significance. Similarly, people are drawn to sports volunteerism as it can often be carried out in the company of friends or other family members. This is especially true in close-knit communities where those families and individuals who volunteer in this way are held in high regard by wider society. Developing this point further, it may be argued that national patriotism can also represent a significant motivating factor for sports volunteers (Bang and Chelladurai 2003). This is especially true in the context of international sporting events. In this setting, an individual may derive particular satisfaction from seeing their country host a sporting event to popular acclaim.

Volunteerism can also help to improve one's mental health and encourage overall levels of well-being amongst a population. In an interesting study conducted in 2008, the Corporation of National and Community Service identified a host of health benefits arising from volunteerism (Corporation for National and Community Service 2007). In fact, the key findings of the study established a correlation between volunteering and greater life satisfaction rates, along with a reduction in anxiety and depression levels. The study also revealed that individuals who reported higher levels of self-esteem, life satisfaction and health levels were more likely to volunteer than those that did not (Thoits and Hewitt 2001). These initial findings are supported by numerous other research papers published in the field, which together confirm that a well-designed volunteer experience enhances feelings of accomplishment and societal contribution (Greenfield and Marks 2004).

Longitudinal research work conducted in the United States has also linked volunteerism with physical health improvements, notably longer lifespans (Musick, Herzog, and House 1999). This is especially apparent amongst older volunteers who benefit from the changes they experience in terms of their role in life and improved social relations (Li and Ferraro 2006). These findings are supported by an earlier study conducted during the 2002 Commonwealth Games staged in England, which considered factors that had motivated the volunteers at that event. Almost all of the volunteers (96%) felt that it would represent a fulfilling experience in terms of contributing to wider society. Moreover, a further 91% agreed that they would gain satisfaction through assisting others, along with being part of a team and presenting the host city of Manchester to an international audience.

The social impact of sports volunteerism

The very essence of voluntary work coheres around the fundamental elements of human experience, which consist of individuals assisting others and, in the process it seems, helping themselves. In modern society, volunteerism can be viewed as a form of civic activism, and seen from that perspective, it again gives rise to a range of positive societal outcomes (Mihajlovic, Komnenic, and Kastratovic 2010). Indeed, one of these is that without such input, there would be a significant reduction in the opportunities available for others to both participate in, and view, sport. As a consequence of this potential decline, it would be expected that the health of the public, amongst other negative outcomes, would decline. Sports' volunteering also affords young people, in particular, the opportunity to be positively engaged in society at the expense of other undesirable and antisocial alternatives.

In the United Kingdom, the concept of using sport to pursue social policy outcomes has been evident since the accession of the New Labour government in the mid-1990s. Unveiling a programme which linked sports volunteerism to desirable outcomes, such as reducing deviance, engaging the disaffected, encouraging educational attainment and upgrading skills and improved employability credentials, was an important component of the party's programme for government in the late 1990s (Social Exclusion Unit 1998; Home Office Citizenship Survey 2005). The underlying potential of sports volunteerism in this regard is also demonstrated within other research, conducted in 2010, which presented evidence that youth volunteering in sport was associated with increased community orientation, improved social awareness, discipline and other positive behavioural adjustments (Kay and Bradbury 2009).

Another key societal advantage attributed to sports volunteerism is its role in the safe-guarding of sports facilities within one's own community. Moreover, successful volunteering programmes can pave the way for additional sports investment, which can again increase participation levels within local settings. Volunteering can also often provide a platform for individuals to participate in 'niche' sports, which may not otherwise be considered as viable investment opportunities for private sector operators (Sports Volunteers in England 2002 2003). Sports volunteerism can further build towards greater social cohesion and integration, especially amongst those emerging from different ethnic backgrounds and nationalities, along with individuals from otherwise divided societies, assisting an overall movement towards positive change and enhanced levels of trust and reciprocity (Eley and Kirk 2002).

The economic impact of sports volunteerism

Thus, the potential of sport to act as a source of economic regeneration and added value has long been accepted (Gratton, Shibli, and Coleman 2005; Misener and Mason 2006). However, the economic contribution of those who volunteer within the industry has, to date, been subject to comparatively limited assessment. A number of reasons are posited for this trend. Again, to confirm a point made earlier, Doherty (2006) underlines the view that only a small number of industrialized countries actually record data on volunteering, thus restricting awareness of its impact within wider society. Studying volunteerism levels across international borders is also often problematical on account of the variations that exist in definitions, methodologies and research that arise when measuring its economic influence. As a result, most of the limited data that are currently available emerge from privately sponsored or commissioned surveys, which deploy small samples, variable definitions and questions and often utilize unreliable methodologies (Lyons, Wijkstrom, and Clary 1998; Rochester 2009; Salamon, Sokolowski, and Haddock 2011).

Despite these complications, a number of studies that have shared similar definitions and methodologies have been conducted. In terms of measuring economic contributions, the principal methodologies include measurement of opportunity cost, replacement cost and contingent valuations (Gratton and Taylor 2000). Replacement cost is often the most commonly applied approaches and measures the value of volunteers by the cost of substituting one hour of paid work for one hour of volunteer work undertaken within a comparable position (Nichols 2003; Mook and Sousa 2005). This places a value on their individual voluntary contribution by considering what it would cost to hire someone to complete the said work in a paid capacity. Of course, this approach assumes that volunteers and paid employees are interchangeable, which is sometimes not entirely appropriate. Indeed, some analysts find this approach controversial as it fails to accept the possibility that a volunteer's skills and experience may differ from those of a specifically recruited paid employee (Abraham and Mackie 2005; Forster 2006).

Opportunity cost is another common assessment approach that measures the value of the time that the volunteer could spend in his or her regular job if he/she were not volunteering. In this context, this method measures the volunteer's contribution with reference to the value of the alternative opportunity they are forgoing in order to carry out their duties (Freeman 1997; Davies 2004). A further methodology is contingent valuation. This technique relies on the stated amount that those making use of a non-market service would be willing to pay for it if it were no longer available to them free of charge. Whilst this approach is highly subjective, some notable economists argue that, utilizing a proper design, this strategy may offer quite reliable indicators of value (Adamowics, Boxall, and Louviere 1998; Mook and Quarter 2003; Quarter, Mook, and Richmond 2003).

Apart from measuring economic input at an individual level, attention must also be placed on the extent of volunteer contribution both at an organizational level and at an macro-economic level. From an organizational perspective, this takes into account the value of the additional activities and services an organization can offer as a result of its voluntary assistance, along with added value that is created through access to new funding sources and improved relations with stakeholders, as well as with the wider community.

Equally as important is the effect of volunteerism at a macro-economic level. Attracting exposure and publicity in this regard is crucial in attaining public policy inclusion and financing. Despite the obvious advantages of volunteerism to any national economy, most countries do not allocate a specific budget to support voluntary work schemes, which is regrettable. In the United Kingdom, for example, sports volunteerism is financed largely by the government along with other public sources, such as that country's national lottery programme (Sport England 2007).

Despite the measurement difficulties that persist, there are some published studies which do highlight the economic returns sports volunteerism can provide. For example, the economic value of sports volunteerism in England was just under £2 billion in 2010 (Sport England 2010). Whilst the sports industry there possesses large-scale private sector investment, this level of return can also be witnessed in other countries, where sport is comprised mainly of smaller, community-based bodies, such as in Northern Ireland. With a population of just over 1.5 million, the economic value of sports volunteers in that country in 2008 was measured at £106 million. This figure is in turn equivalent to 17% of the total sports-related economic activity within that UK region (Volunteer Now 2010).

These figures, ratios and trends can also be witnessed in other parts of the world as well. In a very significant study, Dalziel (2011) conducted research around the economic contribution of volunteers to the sports industry in New Zealand between 2004 and 2009, using the replacement cost method previously outlined. His study found that, on average, sports volunteers in the country provided 51.3 million hours of output per annum. This translated into an overall economic contribution that ranged from NZ$ 704.3 million in 2004 to NZ$ 728 million in 2009. These figures are equitable to the annual total income of the population employed in paid sport in the country, which was NZ$ 875 million (Dalziel 2011).

In a similarly insightful study, Chalip (1999) conducted a predictive research report on the economic valuation of the volunteers at the 2000 Olympic Games in Australia, again utilizing the cost replacement methodology. Prior to the Games, the Sydney Organising Committee recruited 40,000 volunteers who produced a combined output of 5.45 million hours, equating to an economic contribution of A$ 109.75 million. Taking into account the overall cost of recruiting the volunteers (A$ 5.1 million), a relative ratio of 21.52:1 was established; meaning for every dollar invested in the volunteers, an approximate return of A$ 21.52 was realized. This study also suggests that the event, to a significant degree, was made possible thanks to the assistance of the volunteers. Considering that the Games injected an additional A$ 6.5 million of economic activity into the Australian economy, the indirect contribution of the volunteers in this regard is noteworthy (Chalip 1999).

In placing this report into context, it offers an insight into the contribution volunteers can offer in economic terms, especially at large-scale sporting events. For example, the total economic impact of the UK Olympic and Paralympic Games in 2012 was estimated to be in the region of £16.5 billion over a twelve-year period (Lloyds Banking Group 2012). The Games are also anticipated to generate a net increase in the number of tourists to the United Kingdom of £10.8 million with a linked tourist spend of £2 billion in the years ahead. Without the contribution of the 70,000 volunteers who assisted at the event, it would be unlikely that this meeting would have been able to return such impressive economic results. From this perspective, it is apparent just what form of contribution volunteers do actually make, both directly and indirectly, in economic terms.

However, this level of economic contributions is not merely restricted to events of the magnitude and scale of an Olympic Games. Annual sporting events such as Formula 1 racing, which also rely heavily on volunteers, often return impressive economic figures in their own right. For example, the British F1 Grand Prix in 2011 contributed an estimated £14 million to the UK Treasury during that year (Price Waterhouse Coopers 2011). Similar amounts were realized at the Australian Formula 1 Grand Prix in 2005, which created a total expenditure injection of A$51.25 million into the Australian economy (Dwyer, Forsyth, and Spurr 2006). It is appropriate again to highlight that these kinds of economic returns would not be as pronounced were it not for the assistance of the thousands of volunteers who give of their time annually across the Formula 1 calendar.

Sports volunteerism can also contribute, in an economic sense, in a range of ways apart from assisting in the profitability of major sporting events. For example, volunteering can aid the creation of innovative partnerships between businesses, public authorities and voluntary sector organizations. These kinds of partnerships can lead to the creation of new paid employment opportunities for many involved in the voluntary sector. Another indirect economic outcome relates to the concept of 'volunteer tourism'. This term describes a situation where an individual may travel to a certain location beyond their immediate locality to volunteer at a specific event. For example, the London Summer Olympics of 2012 attracted many volunteers from outside the Greater London area. To partake in such events, these volunteers used hotels and spent money in the locality, in much the same way that a tourist would do were they visiting the city to attend the event itself. This creates inward economic migration and enhanced activities in many cities that host large-scale sporting events and commonly attract large numbers of volunteers. This effect can be multiplied by a factor of two or three if a volunteer brings their family or friends to accompany them in fulfilment of their volunteering duties (Addarii, De Amicis, and Flanagan 2011). The economic figures associated with sport volunteering programmes often go unnoticed by public sector authorities internationally. Therefore, it is not entirely surprising that sports volunteerism often remains a missing public policy component, despite its obvious economic and societal benefits.

Motorsport volunteerism and the concept of a social contract

The regulatory system in motorsport promoted by the sport's world governing body, the *Fédération Internationale de l'Automobile* (FIA), is aimed at providing the framework under which sporting competition takes place. It provides the balance of managing the sport in a safe and controlled way, at the same time allowing the competitive nature of those involved to satisfy their need for challenge and excitement. In motorsport, by signing on at the start of an event, volunteers enter into an ethical agreement with the organizers to become their representatives for its duration and to administer the activities of the event. The volunteer officials who manage and administer the sport are also subject to its rules and regulations, in particular in achieving standards of professionalism and behaviour. At all levels, there are processes and procedures to ensure the safety of those involved and especially those who may be working close to the track or rally stage, such as marshals and timing crew. They accept the authority of the organization to set rules and administer sanctions if these are broken, yet there is no obligation to submit to the rule of the organization other than their desire to do so. The question is, does this amount to a social contract in the acknowledged sense?

Social contracts

Social contract theory holds that people's moral and political obligations depend on an agreement or 'contract' amongst them to create the society in which they live. Hobbes, who is considered to be one of the founders of social contract theory, argued in his Leviathan published in 1651 that a mutual exchange of benefits was necessary for the formation of a contract and this is born out in modern-day contract principles. Hobbes, however, concluded that if a person did something for free as a result of self-serving or even altruistic motivations, then this was a gift, not a contract.

Early debates on the subject considered the concept that society consented, rather than had an obligation, to be governed. Rousseau (1762) concludes that 'Each of us puts his person and all his power in common under the supreme direction of the general will, and, in our corporate capacity, we receive each member as an indivisible part of the whole' (23). Rousseau argued that a citizen cannot pursue his true interest by being an egoist but must instead subordinate himself to the law created by the citizenry acting as a collective.

According to him, only by entering into a social contract can man become fully human. In considering how freedom might be considered possible in a civilized society, Rousseau contended that in our natural state, mankind is free of restraints of behaviour and conduct, not governed by rules or regulations. By entering into a social contract, man subjugates himself to the rules and constraints that society considers appropriate to allow him to live and participate in that community, and further, by offering up our physical freedom, we acquire civil freedom allowing society to flourish.

Rousseau proposed that a point in nature is reached, whereby people need to join forces to survive. How this is achieved is by the formation of a 'social contract', in which people come together in agreement on a set of rules and norms, which bind themselves together unconditionally in order to preserve freedom. Rousseau draws three main conclusions from this: (a) because the condition which creates this need is common to all, then they will endeavour to make this as simple as possible for all; (b) because people enter into this contract freely and unconditionally, then the individual does not have rights to stand in opposition to the common will; and (c) that, as no one is set above anyone else, personal freedom is not lost by entering into the social contract.

In *The Second Treatise of Government*, John Locke (1689) explains the nature of legitimate government in terms of natural rights and the social contract. The concept of consent is fundamental to the role of government – that people consent to be governed and that this is the way that political societies are founded. Although people have certain obligations deriving from the laws of nature, obligations of a special nature only occur consensually. Although much of Locke's opinions are founded on the need to protect property, he believes that people are willing to give up their rights to a higher authority in order to achieve protection and order.

The early works of Hobbes, Locke and Rousseau set the foundations for modern social contract theory, although there were some detractors. In 'Of the Original Contract', Hume (1748) described the idea of a 'social contract' as a convenient fiction, arguing that consent of the governed was the 'ideal foundation on which a government could rest' (21).

Modern-day Western contract thinking is based on a will theory, in which a contract is not presumed valid unless all parties agree to it voluntarily and without coercion. This, according to Kary (2000), takes the consent theories of the seventeenth-century theorists to an extreme. A party enters into a modern-day contract knowing all of its terms and conditions and accedes to them as they had decided mutually on what these were. In contrast, social contract theory holds that we are bound by a higher principle that mutual obligation will govern what is considered right and more importance was attached to consideration. In other words, a mutual exchange of benefits was necessary to the creation of a valid contract. Most contracts formed at this time contained implicit, rather than explicit, terms founded on the nature of the contractual relationship between the parties rather than the choices made by them.

In motorsport, the rules of the national governing bodies (ASNs) are in the public domain and accessible to those who engage with them. The duties of motorsport officials are proscribed in the FIA International Sporting Code (Article 11 and Appendix H) and the sanctions and penalties detailed in Article 12. Likewise, the regulations of the ASNs distil these obligations down in each country, but it is unlikely that many of the volunteer marshals below senior official level would prove familiar with any or even some of these. The regulations are of a general nature when they relate specifically to officials. There are obligations of punctuality and performance placed on the volunteers, which require them to be present at the events on time and to remain at their allocated post until the event releases them. Yet, there is no explicit sanction against them if they default on these obligations, other than the disappointment of their peers and, in extreme circumstances, being removed from their position of trust and being denied to the opportunity to volunteer at future events. Likewise, in certain disciplines, performance targets are required to be met to demonstrate competence, such as extrication teams on FIA events, which require the removal of a driver from a vehicle within a set period of time and in a safe manner. Countless hours of training go into meeting this standard which, although required to be achieved to allow the event to continue in a safe way, carries no personal penalty if it is not, other than a perception of failure of the individual or team.

By the act of signing on at the start of an event, the volunteer willingly acquiesces to such rules and obligations, probably without considering their detail but in the belief that the governance arrangements exist in their own interest. This belief could be what forms the social contract between organizers and officials, but on the other hand, the counter argument could be made that those entering into such a contract should take the time to make themselves aware of its conditions, obligations and sanctions before doing so. So does the answer lie elsewhere?

Psychological contracts

Recent needs to understand the volunteer experience has led to an interest in the concept of the psychological contract, which is 'an individual's beliefs regarding the terms and conditions of a reciprocal exchange agreement between that focal person and another party' (Rousseau 1989, 123).

Although psychological contracts were originally defined by Argyris (1960), Levinson (1962) and Schein (1980) to identify the subjectivity of employment relationships, they are commonly used to understand informal relationships between an employer and employee in terms of expectations and disappointments. Considered as describing the individual perceptions created by organizations about what would be exchanged between them and employees in terms of mutual contributions, Morrison and Robinson (1997) argue that to have a psychological contract, a relationship between an individual and an organization must exist and that the individual must have expectations about what he will get from the organization in return. However, we must recognize that expectations are still distinct from a psychological contract as expectations refer simply to what the employee expects to receive from his or her employer (Wanous 1977) and thus are considered un-enforceable. The psychological contract, on the other hand, refers to the perceived mutual obligations that characterize the employee's relationship with their employer (Robinson and Rousseau 1994, 246), which, although not explicit, could be held as supporting contentions in a dispute over employment. The deliberate creation of these expectations by an organization – in promising something in exchange for the individual's efforts – evolves into obligations, and thus, a 'contract' is formed based on this reciprocal arrangement.

When organizations meet their perceived obligations towards employees, then the employees are motivated and prepared to expend effort and be innovative, creative and support management (Rousseau 1990). However, when this relationship breaks down and the expectations are not met, the value of this exchange is diminished and employees tend to lose trust in the management, consequently commitment levels, and thus, contribution, eventually, decreases (Robinson and Rousseau 1994, 247).

Relationships between organizations and employees can be evaluated in the context of the level of exchange they have. This exchange may not necessarily be monetary or materialistic, but the greater the perceived value of the exchange, the stronger the relationship. In terms of motorsport volunteers, where there is no formal employer/employee relationship due to the frequent absence of a written agreement, the concept of the psychological contract considers that this relationship exists in that volunteers accept the authority of the organization and are willing to abide by its rules and regulations. These obligations are not necessarily formalized, but are often imprecise and informal. Nevertheless, the important element in any such arrangement, especially in employment relationships, is that they are believed by the employee to be part of their relationship with the employer and how they are perceived on a practical level. In other words, 'an individual's belief in mutual obligations between that person and another party such as an employer' (Rousseau and Tijoriwala 1998, 679).

The concept of psychological contracts has also been used to explain the attitudes and behaviour of paid employees (Zhao et al. 2007) and is widely applied to the consideration of relationships between employers and employees (Rousseau 1989; Morrison and Robinson 1997; Roehling 1997). Nichols and Ojala (2009, 372) considered that despite the limited research into the application of psychological contracts in the specific area of volunteers (Farmer and Fedor 1999; Liao-Troth 2001; Ralston, Downward, and Lumsdon 2004; Smith 2004; Starnes 2007), there appeared to be considerable potential to offer an understanding in terms of employment without the reward of pay and relate this to mainstream human resource management practices.

In a psychological contract between employee and employer, the contribution that the employee makes towards an organization obligates the organization to do something for the employee in return (Rousseau 1989) and in particular when the organization promises something to the employee before the contribution is made. From an altruistic viewpoint of the volunteer, this expectation may be considerably less in material terms and more in self-benefit and the feeling of making a contribution for the greater good. By volunteering to satisfy certain motives, people also have certain expectations of the experience in terms of self-satisfaction, fulfilment and purpose. It is likely that these expectations will differ from those of the paid employee (Farmer and Fedor 1999; Cullinane and Dundon 2006) who is more likely to be driven by more fundamental needs of employment and security.

Nichols and Ojala (2009, 375) identified that there were clear differences between the expectations of the managers and administrators of sport compared to that of volunteers. The former had considerable expectations in terms of professionalism, regulatory and legal compliance, as well as reliability and commitment. Volunteers focus more on elements such as participation, enjoyment, satisfaction, responsibility, interesting work and challenges, added to which is an expectation of clear and correct communication, good management and a safe environment, together with appreciation and support (Ralston, Downward, and Lumsdon 2004).

Psychological contracts can be either transactional or relational depending on the circumstances (Rousseau 1990; Morrison and Robinson 1997). Transactional contracts tend to involve specific obligations mutually agreed for a short term, such as one-off or special events which do not engender any specific feelings of loyalty (McDonald and Makin 1999). In contrast, relational contracts involve a much longer period of involvement, sometimes over many years, linked with more open-ended and less clearly defined mutual obligations, but with a definite feeling of loyalty and commitment on both parts. The latter is very prevalent in motorsport, which engenders long-term relationships as part of the event team often year after year. Studies surrounding the motivation of event volunteers identify the positive correlation of this to the satisfaction of volunteers with the volunteering experience. Farrell, Johnston, and Twynam (1998) indicate that if motivational needs and thus expectations are met, then volunteers are more likely to return as volunteers for future events.

Bang and Ross (2009) identify that the importance of satisfying volunteer motivations can be explained in terms of self-determination (citing Deci and Ryan 1985a). Autonomy and control are important motivational factors associated with a sense of volition a person's intrinsic interests and goals. Autonomy is positively associated with self-actualization, private self-consciousness, ego development, interest and self-esteem (Deci and Ryan 1985b), whereas controlled orientation is positively related to the external locus of control, private and public self-consciousness, hostility and ego involvement (Deci and Ryan 1985b; Knee, Neighbors, and Vietor 2001; Neighbors, Vietor, and Knee 2002). Accordingly, the satisfaction derived by the volunteer from participation in events will lead them to volunteer for further events as they experience psychological need satisfaction as a result. In addition, the positive feeling of satisfaction experienced by a volunteer may encourage a longer-term commitment to the organization.

Paid vs. unpaid?

Lockstone-Binney et al. (2010) argue that as volunteers are unpaid there is a 'different psychological contract between them and the organization in which they work in comparison with formally remunerated staff' (citing Handy (1988); Kim et al. (2009). Wilson (1997) considers volunteer work as 'unpaid work provided to parties to whom the worker owes no contractual, familial or friendship obligations'. Volunteers often do exactly the same work as paid workers, the difference being the absence of a wage.

Vroom (1964) considered motivation as 'a process governing choices amongst alternative forms of voluntary activities, a process controlled by the individual'. Individuals make choices based on their prediction of the outcome and whether that behaviour will match or achieve the desired result or reward. Motivation is derived from a person's expectancy that a given action or effort will produce a certain result and the desirability of that outcome is known as 'valence'. Porter and Lawler (1968) concluded that a person's motivation to complete a task is affected by the reward they expect to receive for completing the task. However, Porter and Lawler introduced further dimensions to Vroom's expectancy theory, categorizing the reward into intrinsic rewards, which are 'the positive feelings that come from completing the task eg satisfaction, sense of achievement', and extrinsic rewards, which emanate externally (eg bonuses, commissions and pay increases).

The exchange of monetary reward for labour in the context of motorsport is largely irrelevant as the reward is taken in other ways. Social rewards such as interaction with other like-minded people, training and development of skills not normally related to or usually available in the workplace and satisfaction from a number of factors all constitute a form of reward that can be exchanged.

Rochester (2006) noted that whilst it is usually held that volunteers should not be out of pocket as a result of their involvement and should not receive any other material reward, this is not necessarily the universal practice. According to Blacksell and Phillips (1994), their study of volunteers revealed that a significant number of respondents had received some kind of consideration over and above the reimbursement of expenses. The availability of guest tickets to major events within the sport, free accommodation, meals and so on could be seen as blurring the boundaries of what is acceptable 'fringe benefits' and what is material reward, going beyond the realms of pure volunteering. However, it could also be argued that such privileges are merely recognition thanks for the efforts of the volunteer. In contrast, it may be noted that volunteers often incurred personal expenses in the course of their volunteer activities and that whilst employees would normally expect to receive reimbursement, volunteers often did not or were unaware that they were entitled to do so. In a survey of British marshals, it was found that the overwhelming interest of marshals was recognition for their efforts, followed by meal vouches and a guaranteed finishing time. There was a strong reaction against getting paid as it was thought by respondents that this would detract from the quality of marshals.

Cnaan, Handy, and Wadsworth (1996) held that the term 'volunteer' is used widely to describe non-salaried service. They attempted to 'delineate the boundaries of the term volunteer' and identified four key dimensions commonly found in most definitions of volunteer (free choice, remuneration, structure and beneficiaries). These dimensions indicate that the act of volunteering is not normally done out of any obligation to do so, more out of a willingness or motivation to do so. The purity of the volunteering act is in their opinion dependent on the net cost to the volunteer (375).

Common to all, however, appears to be a willingness of volunteers to exchange work in return for perceived benefits or a wage-work bargain without the 'wage'. Cnaan expresses this as a continuum with free choice ranging from 'free will' to an 'obligation to volunteer' and remuneration from 'none at all' to 'stipend or low pay'. They proposed an internal continuum for each dimension that distinguished between 'pure' and 'broadly defined' volunteers.

Conclusion

Discretionary behaviour, or that not recognized by the formal reward system, can be traced back to the work of Barnard (1938) and Katz (1964). Organ (1988, 4) in describing organizational citizenship behaviour (OCB) said that it 'represents individual behaviour that is discretionary, not directly or explicitly recognized by the formal reward system, and in the aggregate promotes the efficient and effective functioning of the organization'. Although this created considerable debate and criticism, especially to the altruistic aspects of the concept (Organ 1997), could this idea of discretionary behaviour also be used to consider this paradigm? Certainly, in considering the concept of a social contract as a construct of motorsport volunteerism, the discretionary behaviour element is fundamental to the willingness to be governed.

The question of volunteerism specifically as a social contract can offer some insight into the motives of volunteers and their acquiescence to the governance of the sporting authority. How far this explains motivation is limited, but probably forms part of the overall picture. The extent to which a motorsport marshal knowingly enters into such a contract in full appreciation of its terms is not clear and would need to be explored in much greater detail than has been done to date.

In general, the consideration of the concept of a psychological contract of volunteers has adapted approaches from studies of paid employees and has not extensively explored the psychological contract as socially constructed. Given that there is a general recognition of the enormous contribution made to motorsport by volunteers, it is important that a consolidated understanding of their motivation is developed, not just in terms of particular and discrete theories. An individual's volunteer motivation reflects (i) the actualization and continuity of voluntary activity from both a theoretical and a practical perspective (ii) the sociological notion of future commitment and participation (Yeung 2004). In particular, when it comes to the matters of recruitment and retention, this understanding is fundamental to the success and future prosperity of motorsport.

Disclosure statement

No potential conflict of interest was reported by the authors.

References

Abraham, K. G., and C. Mackie. 2005. *Beyond the Market: Designing Non-market Accounts for the United States*. Washington, DC: The National Academies Press.

Adamowics, W., P. Boxall, and J. Louviere. 1998. "Stated Preference Approaches for Measuring Passive Use Values: Choice Experiments and Contingency Valuation." *American Journal of Agricultural Economics* 80 (1): 64–75. doi:10.2307/3180269.

Addarii, F., L. De Amicis, and T. Flanagan. 2011. "The Economic Value of Volunteering and Contribution in Kind." Brussels Roundtable Discussion.

Argyris, C. 1960. *Understanding Organizational Behaviour*. Homewood, IL: Dorsey.

Auld, C. J., and G. Cuskelly. 2001. "Behavioral Characteristics of Volunteers: Implications for Community Sport and Recreation Organisations." *Australian Parks and Leisure* 4 (2): 29–37.

Australian Bureau of Statistics. 2012. "Volunteers in Sport." Accessed April 15, 2013. http://www.abs. gov.au/ausstats/abs@.nsf/Products/4156.0~2012~Chapter~Volunteers+in+Sport?OpenDocument

Bang, H., and P. Chelladurai. 2003. "Motivation and Satisfaction in Volunteering for 2002 World Cup in Korea." Paper Presented at the Conference of the North American Society for Sport Management. Ithaca, NY.

Bang, H., and S. D. Ross. 2009. "Volunteer Motivation and Satisfaction." *Journal of Venue and Event Management* 1: 61–77.

Barnard, C. 1938. *The Functions of the Executive*. Cambridge, MA: Harvard University Press.

Blacksell, S., and D. Phillips. 1994. *Paid to Volunteer; the Extent of Paying Volunteers in the 1990s*. London: Volunteer Centre UK.

Chalip, L. 1999. "Volunteers and the Organisation of the Olympic Games: Economic and Formative Aspects." Accessed April 17, 2013. http://olympicstudies.uab.es/volunteers/chapil.html

Cnaan, R. A., F. Handy, and M. Wadsworth. 1996. "Defining Who is a Volunteer: Conceptual and Empirical Considerations." *Nonprofit and Voluntary Sector Quarterly* 25 (3): 364–383. doi:10.1177/0899764096253006.

CNN Corporation. 2010. "World Cup to the Olympics: Eight Sports Volunteering Opportunities." Accessed April 13, 2013. http://www.cnn.co.uk/2010/TRAVEL/06/10/sport.volunteers/index.html

Corporation for National and Community Service. 2007. *The Health Benefits of Volunteering*. Washington, DC. Accessed April 15, 2013. http://www.nationalservice.gov/sites/default/files/documents/07_0506_hbr.pdf

Cullinane, N., and T. Dundon. 2006. "The Psychological Contract: A Critical Review." *International Journal of Management Reviews* 8 (2): 113–129. doi:10.1111/ijmr.2006.8.issue-2.

Dalziel, P. 2011. "The Economic and Social Value of Sport and Recreation in New Zealand." Research report number 322. Accessed April 15, 2013. researcharchive.lincoln.ac.nz/dspace/bitstream/10182/.../aeru_rr_322.pdf

Davies, L. 2004. "Valuing the Voluntary Sector in Sport: Rethinking Economic Analysis." *Leisure Studies* 23 (4): 347–364. doi:10.1080/0261436042000209146.

Deci, E. L., and R. M. Ryan. 1985a. *Intrinsic Motivation and Self-determination in Human Behaviour*. New York: Plenum Press.

Deci, E. L., and R. M. Ryan. 1985b. "The General Causality Orientations Scale: Self-determination in Personality." *Journal of Research in Personality* 19 (2): 109–134. doi:10.1016/0092-6566(85)90023-6.

Doherty, A. 2006. "Sport Volunteerism: An Introduction to This Special Issue." *Sport Management Review* 9: 105–109. doi:10.1016/S1441-3523(06)70021-3.

Dwyer, L., P. Forsyth, and R. Spurr. 2006. "Economic Impact of Sport Events: A Reassessment." *Tourism Review International* 10 (4): 207–216. doi:10.3727/154427206779367118.

Eley, D., and D. Kirk. 2002. "Developing Citizenship through Sport: The Impact of a Sport-based Volunteer Programme on Young Sport Leaders." *Sport, Education and Society* 7 (2): 151–166. doi:10.1080/1357332022000018841.

Farmer, S. M., and D. B. Fedor. 1999. "Volunteer Participation and Withdrawal." *Nonprofit Management and Leadership* 9 (4): 349–368. doi:10.1002/(ISSN)1542-7854.

Farrell, J. M., M. E. Johnston, and D. G. Twynam. 1998. "Volunteer Motivation, Satisfaction, and Management at an Elite Sporting Competition." *Journal of Sport Management* 12 (4): 288–300. doi:10.1123/jsm.12.4.288.

Forster, J. 2006. "Global Sports Organisations and Their Governance." *Corporate Governance* 6 (1): 72–83. doi:10.1108/14720700610649481.

Freeman, R. 1997. "Working for Nothing: The Supply of Volunteer Labour." *Journal of Labor Economics* 15 (1): S140–S166. doi:10.1086/209859.

Giannoulakis, C., C. Wang, and D. Gray. 2008. "Measuring Volunteer Motivation in Mega Sporting Events." *Journal of Event Management* 11 (2): 191–200.

Gratton, C., S. Shibli, and R. Coleman. 2005. "Sport and Economic Regeneration in Cities." *Urban Studies* 42 (5–6): 985–999. doi:10.1080/00420980500107045.

Gratton, C., and P. Taylor. 2000. *The Economics of Sport and Recreation: An Economic Analysis*. 2nd ed. London: Routledge.

Green, B., and L. Chalip. 1998. "Sports Volunteers: Research Agenda and Application." *Sports Marketing Quarterly* 7 (2): 14–23.

Greenfield, E., and N. Marks. 2004. "Formal Volunteering as a Protective Factor for Older Adults' Psychological Well-being." *The Journals of Gerontology* 59 (5): 27–39.

Handy, C. 1988. *Understanding Voluntary Organizations*. London: Penguin.

Hobbes, Thomas. 1651. *Leviathan*. Edited by C. B. Macpherson. London: Penguin Books. (1985).

Home Office Citizenship Survey. 2005. London: National Centre for Social Research.

Hume, D. 1748. "Of the Original Contract." Part 2, Essay 13; *The Constitution Society*, edited by J. Roland.

Irish Sport Council. 2007. *Irish Sports Monitor*. Dublin.

Kary, J. 2000. "Contract Law and the Social Contract: What Legal History Can Teach Us about the Political Theory of Hobbes and Locke." *Ottawa Law Review* 73 (2): 67–80.

Katz, D. 1964. "The Motivational Basis of Organizational Behavior." *Behavioral Science* 9 (2): 131–146. doi:10.1002/(ISSN)1099-1743.

Kay, T., and S. Bradbury. 2009. "Youth Sport Volunteering: Developing Social Capital?" *Sport, Education and Society* 14 (1): 121–140. doi:10.1080/13573320802615288.

Kim, M., G. T. Trail, J. Lim, and Y. K. Kim. 2009. "The Role of Psychological Contract in Intention to Continue Volunteering." *Journal of Sport Management* 23 (5): 549–573. doi:10.1123/jsm.23.5.549.

Knee, C. R., C. Neighbors, and N. Vietor. 2001. "Self-determination Theory as a Framework for Understanding Road Rage." *Journal of Applied Social Psychology* 31 (5): 889–904. doi:10.1111/jasp.2001.31.issue-5.

Levinson, H. 1962. *Men, Management and Mental Health*. Cambridge, MA: Harvard University Press.

Li, Y., and K. Ferraro. 2006. "Volunteering in Middle and Later Life: Is Health a Benefit, Barrier or Both?" *Social Forces* 85 (1): 497–519. doi:10.1353/sof.2006.0132.

Liao-Troth, M. A. 2001. "Attitude Differences between Paid Workers and Volunteers." *Non-Profit Management and Leadership* 11 (4): 423–442. doi:10.1002/(ISSN)1542-7854.

Lloyds Banking Group. 2012. "The Economic Impact of the London 2012 Olympic and Paralympic Games." Oxford Economics. Accessed April 17, 2013. http://www.lloydsbankinggroup.com/media/pdfs/lbg/2012/Eco_impact_report.pdf

Locke, John. 1689. *Two Treatises of Government*. Edited by P. Laslett. Cambridge: Cambridge University Press, 1988.

Lockstone-Binney, L., K. Holmes, K. Smith, and T. G. Baum. 2010. "Volunteers and Volunteering in Leisure: Social Science Perspectives." *Leisure Studies* 29 (4): 435–455. doi:10.1080/02614367.2010.527357.

Lunn, P., and R. Layte. 2009. "The Irish Sports Monitor." 3rd Annual Report. The Economic and Social Research Institute. Accessed April 15, 2013. http://www.cavansportspartnership.ie/file/Irish%20Sports%20Monitor%20Report%202009.pdf

Lyons, M., P. Wijkstrom, and G. Clary. 1998. "Comparative Studies of Volunteering: What is Being Studied?" *Voluntary Action* 1 (1): 45–54.

McDonald, D. J., and P. J. Makin. 1999. "The Psychological Contract, Organisational Commitment and Job Satisfaction of Temporary Staff." *Leadership & Organization Development Journal* 21 (2): 84–91. doi:10.1108/01437730010318174.

Mihajlovic, M., N. Komnenic, and E. Kastratovic. 2010. "Volunteers in Sports Organisations." *Sports Management International Journal* 6 (2): 5–18.

Misener, L., and D. S. Mason. 2006. "Creating Community Networks: Can Sporting Events Offer Meaningful Sources of Social Capital?" *Managing Leisure* 11 (1): 39–56. doi:10.1080/13606710500445676.

Mook, L., and J. Quarter. 2003. *How to Assign a Monetary Value to Volunteer Contributions*. Canada: Knowledge Development Centre, Canadian Centre for Philanthropy.

Mook, L., and J. Sousa. 2005. "Accounting for the Value of Volunteer Contributions." *Non-Profit Management and Leadership* 15 (4): 401–415. doi:10.1002/(ISSN)1542-7854.

Morrison, E. W., and S. L. Robinson. 1997. "When Employees Feel Betrayed: A Model of How Psychological Contract Violation Develops." *Academy of Management Review* 22 (1): 226–256. doi:10.2307/259230.

Musick, M., A. Herzog, and J. S. House. 1999. "Volunteering and Mortality among Older Adults: Findings from a National Sample." *Journal of Gerontology, Series B: Psychological Sciences and Social Sciences* 54 (3): 12–19.

Neighbors, C., N. A. Vietor, and C. R. Knee. 2002. "A Motivational Model of Driving Anger and Aggression." *Personality and Social Psychology Bulletin* 28 (3): 324–335. doi:10.1177/0146167202286004.

Nichols, G. 2003. *Volunteers in Sport*. Eastbourne: Leisure Studies Association.

Nichols, G., and E. Ojala. 2009. "Understanding the Management of Sports Events Volunteers through Psychological Contract Theory." *International Journal of Voluntary and Nonprofit Organizations* 20: 369–387. doi:10.1007/s11266-009-9097-9.

Omoto, A., and M. Snyder. 2002. "Considerations of Community: The Context and Process of Volunteerism." *American Behavioral Scientist* 45 (5): 846–867. doi:10.1177/0002764202045005007.

Organ, D. W. 1988. *Organizational Citizenship Behavior: The Good Soldier Syndrome*. Lexington, MA: Lexington Books.

Organ, D. W. 1997. "Organizational Citizenship Behavior: It's Construct Clean-up Time." *Human Performance* 10 (2): 85–97. doi:10.1207/s15327043hup1002_2.

Porter, L. W., and E. E. Lawler. 1968. *Managerial Attitudes and Performance*. Homewood, IL: Richard D. Irwin Inc.

Price Water Coopers. 2011. "Attendances Rise at UK's Biggest Annual Sporting Events." Press Release Issued 04/08/11.

Quarter, J., L. Mook, and B. J. Richmond. 2003. *What Counts: Social Accounting for Non-profits and Cooperatives*. Upper Saddle River, NJ: Prentice Hall.

Ralston, R., P. Downward, and L. Lumsdon. 2004. "The Expectations of Volunteers Prior to the XVII Commonwealth Games, 2002: A Qualitative Study." *Event Management* 9 (1–2): 13–26. doi:10.3727/1525995042781084.

Robinson, S. L., and D. M. Rousseau. 1994. "Violating the Psychological Contract: Not the Exception but the Norm." *Journal of Organizational Behavior* 15 (3): 245–259. doi:10.1002/(ISSN)1099-1379.

Rochester, C. 2006. *Making Sense of Volunteering: A Literature Review*. London: The Commission on the Future of Volunteering, Volunteering England. 1–39.

Rochester, C. 2009. *A Gateway to Work: The Role of Volunteer Centres in Supporting the Link between Volunteering and Employability*. London: IVR.

Roehling, M. V. 1997. "The Origins and Early Development of the Psychological Contract Construct." *Journal of Management History* 3 (2): 204–217. doi:10.1108/13552529710171993.

Rousseau, J.-J. 1762. *The Social Contract and Discourses*. The Constitution Society.

Rousseau, D. M. 1989. "Psychological and Implied Contracts in Organizations." *Employee Responsibilities and Rights Journal* 2 (2): 121–139. doi:10.1007/BF01384942.

Rousseau, D. M. 1990. "New Hire Perceptions of Their Own and Their Employer's Obligations: A Study of Psychological Contracts." *Journal of Organizational Behavior* 11 (5): 389–400. doi:10.1002/(ISSN)1099-1379.

Rousseau, D. M., and S. A. Tijoriwala. 1998. "Assessing Psychological Contracts: Issues, Alternatives and Measures." *Journal of Organizational Behavior* 19 (1): 679–695. doi:10.1002/(SICI)1099-1379(1998)19:1+<679::AID-JOB971>3.0.CO;2-N.

Salamon, L., W. Sokolowski, and M. Haddock. 2011. "Measuring the Economic Value of Volunteer Work Globally: Concepts, Estimates and a Roadmap to the Future." *Ciriec International* 82 (3): 1–10. Accessed April 16, 2013. http://ccss.jhu.edu/wp-content/uploads/downloads/2011/10/Annals-Septmeber-2011.pdf

Schein, E. H. 1980. *Organizational Psychology*. Englewood Cliffs, NJ: Prentice Hall.

Smith, J. 2004. "What They Really Want: Assessing Psychological Contracts of Volunteers." *Journal of Volunteer Administration* 22 (1): 18–21.

Social Exclusion Unit. 1998. *Bringing Britain Together: A National Strategy for Neighbourhood Renewal*. London: Stationery Office.

Sport England. 2007. *Active People Survey – 2*. London: Sport Volunteering.

Sport England. 2010. *Active People Survey – 4*. London: Sport Volunteering.

Sports Volunteers in England 2002. 2003. *A Report for Sport England*. Sheffield: Leisure Industries Research Centre.

Starnes, B. J. 2007. "An Analysis of Psychological Contracts in Volunteerism and the Effect of Contract Breach on Volunteer Contributions to the Organization." *The International Journal of Volunteer Administration* 24 (3): 31–41.

Statistics Canada. 2010. Study: Volunteering in Canada 2010. Accessed April 15, 2013. http://www.statcan.gc.ca/daily-quotidien/120416/dq120416b-eng.pdf

The Executive Board of the United Nations Development Programme. 2013. The United Nations Population Fund and Office for Projects Services New York (2013). Accessed April 12, 2013. www.undp.org/content/dam/undp/library/corporate/.../dp2013-34.doc

Thoits, P., and L. Hewitt. 2001. "Volunteer Work and Well-being." *Journal of Health and Social Behavior* 42 (2): 115–131. doi:10.2307/3090173.

Vancouver Olympics Commission. 2010. "Staging the Olympic Winter Games Knowledge Report." Accessed April 14, 2013. http://www.la84foundation.org/6oic/OfficialReports/2010/2010v2.pdf

Volunteer Now. 2010. "*The Impact of Volunteering in Northern Ireland*." Accessed April 17, 2013. http://www.volunteernow.co.uk/fs/doc/FinalImpactofVolunteeringinSport.pdf

Vroom, V. H. 1964. *Work and Motivation*. New York: Wiley.

Wanous, J. P. 1977. "Organizational Entry: Newcomers Moving from outside to inside." *Psychological Bulletin* 84 (4): 601–618. doi:10.1037/0033-2909.84.4.601.

Wilson, J. 1997. "Who Cares? Toward an Integrated Theory of Volunteer Work." *American Sociological Review* 62 (5): 24–32.

Yeung, A. B. 2004. "The Octagon Model of Volunteer Motivation: Results of a Phenomenological Analysis." *VOLUNTAS: International Journal of Voluntary and Nonprofit Organizations* 15 (1): 21–46. doi:10.1023/B:VOLU.0000023632.89728.ff.

Zakus, D. H., J. Skinner, and A. Edwards. 2009. "Social Capital in Australian Sport." *Sport in Society* 12 (7): 9–20. doi:10.1080/17430430903053224.

Zhao, H., S. J. Wayne, B. C. Glibkowski, and J. Bravo. 2007. "The Impact of Psychological Contract Breach on Work-related Outcomes: A Meta-analysis." *Personnel Psychology* 60 (3): 647–680. doi:10.1111/peps.2007.60.issue-3.

Index